SUPER THIN

THE SUPERWARRIOR GUIDE TO OPTIMUM WEIGHT LOSS

K Abhishek Reddy

K Mahesh Reddy, MD

DISCLAIMER

Every effort has been made to ensure that the information contained in this book is complete and accurate. However, neither the publisher nor the authors are engaged in rendering professional advice or services to the individual reader. The ideas, procedures and suggestions contained in this book are not intended as a substitute for consulting with your physician. All matters regarding your health require medical supervision. This book is intended to supplement, not replace, the advice of a trained health professional. If you know or suspect you have a health problem, you should consult a health professional. The authors and publisher specifically disclaim any liability, loss, or risk, personal and otherwise, that is incurred as a consequence, directly or indirectly, of the use and application of any of the contents of this book.

While the authors have made every effort to provide accurate information, addresses and other contact information at the time of publication, neither the publisher nor the authors assume any responsibility for errors or changes that have occurred. Further, neither the publisher nor the authors have any control over and do not assume any responsibility for third party websites or their websites and content.

Name: Reddy, Abhishek, K, Author; Reddy, Mahesh, K, MD

Title: SUPER THIN / K Abhishek Reddy, K Mahesh Reddy, MD

Description: First Edition

Subjects: Weight-Medicine-Surgery-Health & Fitness-Science

Paperback ISBN: As Imprinted-Affixed-Stated on Print and/or Electronic Versions

Hardcover ISBN: As Imprinted-Affixed-Stated on Print and/or Electronic Versions

E-Book ISBN: As Imprinted-Affixed-Stated on Print and/or Electronic Versions or Not Applicable

DEDICATION

Dedicated to our loving families who have always supported us fully. God Bless.

CONTENTS

INTRODUCTION

Weight Disorders (WD) are complex, multifaceted conditions. They are widely prevalent in our societies. These are a significant problem affecting over 250 million people in America and over 3 billion people worldwide. These cause untold hardship and misery. These have many forms and affect everyone differently. Solutions for this are necessarily going to be multifaceted. These affect men and women. These affect rich and poor. These affect kids and adults. We all may know someone who is suffering from these conditions.

Professionals in different disciplines are trying hard to help. Unfortunately, there is a lot of ignorance clouding this topic across the spectrum. There are conflicting opinions. People are understandably confused about this scourge.

Knowledge on both sides of the spectrum is imperative. It is invaluable in looking at the totality and then endeavoring to mitigate these smartly. This book attempts to strengthen the knowledge base on both sides of the spectrum for optimal healing.

These afflictions can be physical or psychological, spiritual or multi-dimensional causing marked pathological states. It markedly affects and changes our lives. Many lives are tragically shortened both in quality and length. These destroy lives and relationships. They can be managed or cured. Therein lays the promise.

These can be handled in many ways. The particular circumstances of each individual necessitate an individualized action plan. Freedom is about affirming life. If we live, we love. To do this, we need to know more about these disorders, know what causes them and makes them go on. We need to understand. We understand, we know. We know, we solve. We solve, we attenuate or relieve them. Knowledge is power.

Our objectives in writing this book were to share our perspectives and start a journey together where we can understand problems fully. Once we seek, we are empowered to ask more to really understand what may be affecting us. We have tried to give everyone an in depth view of the problems. We have illustrated and described extensively the anatomy, physiology and working details of our bodies. We have identified and clarified the generators and pathologies. We have enumerated diagnostic modalities. We have explained and clarified treatment protocols. This book is neither expected to have the last word on this topic nor be the end all. This gives us the core knowledge of processes affecting discrete body parts or the whole so we can think through the problems and solve them in a smart, logical manner. Any problem can be analyzed. Any problem can be solved. Together, let's do it well.

We are all SuperWarriors at heart. We stand up and fight daily for ourselves, our families, our friends and our societies to the best of our strengths and abilities. SuperWarriors analyze threats, plan and implement realistic, need based solutions. SuperWarriors strive to win, whatever the odds are. Let's free up the inner SuperWarrior in us so we can strategize, fight and win our battles well.

Weight Disorders are a massive societal problem. Let's delineate the problems fully. Let's analyze the problems fully. Let's solve the problems smartly. Together, let's do it well. God Bless.

THE SUPER THIN QUESTIONNAIRE

1. On a scale of 1 through 10, 0 being no weight issues and 10 being
    the worst, how would you grade your weight issues?

    Add 10 points if you have 0/10 scores
    Add 7.5 points if you have 1-3/10 scores
    Add 5 points if you have 4-7/10 scores
    Add 2.5 points if you have 8-10/10 scores

2. On a scale of 1 through 10, 0 being the best and 10 being the
    worst how would you grade your body image issues?

    Add 10 points if you have 0/10 scores
    Add 7.5 points if you have 1-3/10 scores
    Add 5 points if you have 4-7/10 scores
    Add 2.5 points if you have 8-10/10 scores

3. On a scale of 1 through 10, 0 being the least stress and 10 being
    the worst, how would you grade your stress level?

    Add 10 points if you have 0/10 scores
    Add 7.5 points if you have 1-3/10 scores
    Add 5 points if you have 4-7/10 scores
    Add 2.5 points if you have 8-10/10 scores

4. On a scale of 1 through 10, 0 being the least depression and 10 being the worst, how would you grade your depression level?

   Add 10 points if you have 0/10 scores
   Add 7.5 points if you have 1-3/10 scores
   Add 5 points if you have 4-7/10 scores
   Add 2.5 points if you have 8-10/10 scores

5. On a scale of 1 through 10, 0 being the least happiness and 10 being the most, how would you grade your happiness level?

   Add 10 points if you have 8-10/10 scores
   Add 7.5 points if you have 4-7/10 scores
   Add 5 points if you have 1-3/10 scores
   Add 2.5 points if you have 0/10 scores

6. On a scale of 1 through 10, 0 being the least fit and 10 being the most, how would you grade your fitness level?

   Add 10 points if you have 8-10/10 scores
   Add 7.5 points if you have 4-7/10 scores
   Add 5 points if you have 1-3/10 scores
   Add 2.5 points if you have 0/10 scores

7. On a scale of 1 through 10, 0 being the least sociable and 10 being the most, how would you grade your sociability level?

   Add 10 points if you have 8-10/10 scores
   Add 7.5 points if you have 4-7/10 scores
   Add 5 points if you have 1-3/10 scores
   Add 2.5 points if you have 0/10 scores

8. On a scale of 1 through 10, 0 being the least loving and 10 being the most, how would you grade your love scale?

   Add 10 points if you have 8-10/10 scores
   Add 7.5 points if you have 4-7/10 scores
   Add 5 points if you have 1-3/10 scores
   Add 2.5 points if you have 0/10 scores

9. On a scale of 1 through 10, 0 being the least sleep adequacy and 10 being the most, how would you grade your sleep level?

    Add 10 points if you have 8-10/10 scores
    Add 7.5 points if you have 4-7/10 scores
    Add 5 points if you have 1-3/10 scores
    Add 2.5 points if you have 0/10 scores

10. On a scale of 1 through 10, 0 being the least sexual activity and 10 being the most, how would you grade your sexuality level?

    Add 10 points if you have 8-10/10 scores
    Add 7.5 points if you have 4-7/10 scores
    Add 5 points if you have 1-3/10 scores
    Add 2.5 points if you have 0/10 scores

Please add all the numbers together. Let's then go to the scoring system and see where it takes us. We can see where we are at and this may point us to a more promising and rewarding future.

SCORE

75-100: Minimal to mild issues, you are mainly issue free, happy and involved in life. Congratulations. Continue the good work. There are a few things in your life that you could work on that would make it exceptional.

50-75: Mild to moderate issues: You have some issues. You are active in life though these problems can slow you down. Smile, these are fixable. Let's get to work fixing these so you sail smoothly on the ship of life.

25-50: Moderate to marked issues: you have pretty sizable issues. You have significant issues that need to be looked at. Your life is moderately to severely impacted. Well, let's try to fix the problems so you can enjoy life more.

0-25: Marked to severe issues: You are in marked distress. It profoundly affects the quality of your life. We need to fix things up and make it as right as we can. Damn the torpedoes, Full steam ahead.

Now, let's get on to meatier and juicier stuff.

THE CODE OF THE SUPERWARRIOR

As SuperWarriors, we take care of ourselves at all times.

SuperWarriors focus on plenty and abundance.

SuperWarriors do not focus on scarcity or deprivation.

SuperWarriors are grateful for their lives, their families and their gifts.

SuperWarriors expect and get the best of everything.

SuperWarriors lead. When they work together, they think, plan and implement a plan of action to win.

SuperWarriors tend to stay in a prime physical, mental and psychological state.

SuperWarriors are stable, serious and smart.

SuperWarriors stick to a code of honor.

SuperWarriors stand by their word or promise.

SuperWarriors take care of their families, the needy and society.

SuperWarriors take care of their physical, physiological and mental strength.

SuperWarriors are focused, pragmatic and focused.

SuperWarriors look to the future.

SuperWarriors stay in the present while not getting needlessly stuck in the past or the future.

SuperWarriors follow the path of the dharma or the way.

SuperWarriors neither believe in good nor bad or in absolutes of any kind. Life is all relative.

SuperWarriors are calm, relaxed and stay in the moment.

SuperWarriors listen to themselves and do what seems best to them.

SuperWarriors train themselves in body, spirit and mind continually.

SuperWarriors train themselves to serve their communities, neighborhoods, countries and the world in any way they can.

SuperWarriors believe no action is too small or insignificant.

SuperWarriors believe in "Nishkama Karma" Ceaseless action without desire.

SuperWarriors live a simple, full, rich life.

SuperWarriors share what they are blessed with.

SuperWarriors are not attached to material objects or needless pursuits.

SuperWarriors believe in a higher purpose, a supreme being, the universe, controlling power and/or god. It's all the same seamless entity or power.

SuperWarriors are never senseless or delirious when winning.

SuperWarriors are never dispirited when losing. Winning and losing are two sides of the same coin.

SuperWarriors transcend both the opposites.

SuperWarriors take care of their responsibilities and obligations in real time.

SuperWarriors do not get knocked down by adversity. They roll with it and always come out on top.

SuperWarriors turn adversity into triumph.

SuperWarriors turn every situation into a learning opportunity, whether it is good or bad.

SuperWarriors learn from the past but plan for the future while being fully aware in the present.

SuperWarriors regularly assess their skills, weaknesses, opportunities and threats at all times.

SuperWarriors plan, prepare and act decisively.

SuperWarriors expect and get the best out of life.

SuperWarriors are indomitable.

SuperWarriors never give up, whatever the odds.

SuperWarriors are not addicted or dependant on substances, behaviors or experiences.

SuperWarriors analyze and control their thoughts. Your thoughts control your life and your destiny. Your destiny controls your future.

SuperWarriors think independently. They are not easily influenced by fads or cads. Think!

SuperWarriors are grateful for what they have, not what they think they need to have to be happy. Be thankful.

SuperWarriors train their minds, bodies and spirits constantly to be in top fettle. Like your weapon or sword, your body and mind needs to be in top fettle. Stay nimble, smart and strong.

SuperWarriors keep learning and improving in all fields.

SuperWarriors are tolerant and respectful of all people, cultures and religions.

SuperWarriors train smartly for work and play. It's good to be well prepared.

SuperWarriors connect with the earth, the universe and a higher power.

SuperWarriors do not pollute and work to make our earth and universe a better place.

SuperWarriors make their mind and body their closest friends. Always take good care of both these gifts.

SuperWarriors invest time in quality relationships, family and society.

SuperWarriors continually improve the situations and places they are in.

SuperWarriors do not hold on to pain, suffering or trauma.

SuperWarriors appreciate the beauty all around us in the universe.

SuperWarriors welcome love and kindness in their families all the time.

SuperWarriors appreciate the beauty in life.

SuperWarriors live in grace.

SuperWarriors strive to live in truth.

SuperWarriors strive completely to win, irrespective of the odds.

SuperWarriors think not of winning or failure, but about the battle or war.

SuperWarriors Love to Win.

Winning Is Everything.

Winning Is the Only Thing.

***

Neither Pleasure nor Pain
Neither Desire nor Desirelessness
Neither Love nor Hate
Neither Praise nor Blame
Neither Honor nor Dishonor
Neither Liking nor Hating
Renouncing Everything
We Embrace God

***

WHAT ARE WEIGHT DISORDERS?

For scientific and clinical purposes, Weight Disorders (WD) are conditions affecting the human body with disordered body weight and/or body fat and/or anatomic, physiologic, psychological or functional anomalies.

WHAT IS THE SCIENCE BEHIND WEIGHT DISORDERS?

One of the commonest indicators used in determining obesity is via the Body Mass Index (BMI). This measures adiposity or fat mass. This is widely used in exercise, dietary and medical decision making. Many calculators are available to determine this and a few are given in the Resource Guide.

$$BMI = M/H^2$$

BMI Body Mass Index

M Weight

H Height

18-25: Normal Weight

25-30: Overweight

> 30: Obesity

Check with your healthcare provider for additional information as needed regarding BMI, Body fat estimates, etc.

Asian populations like the Japanese and Chinese use lesser BMI values for obesity. Check with your healthcare provider for additional information.

Children have different calculations based on age and sex, obesity is defined as BMI greater than the 95th percentile. Check with your healthcare provider for additional information.

Basal-Standard-Resting Metabolic Rates are indices of energy expenditure which measure our metabolism and rate of energy usage. They usually comprise around two thirds of our daily caloric expenditure and typically decline with each passing decade. Lean body mass is directly correlated with our caloric expenditure and resulting weight. These rates are measured by direct or indirect calorimetry, Harris-Benedict equations, Mifflin St Jeor equation, Katch-McArdle formula, available calculators, etc. These metabolic rates are mainly controlled by the hypothalamus. Optimizing both our metabolic rate and metabolic efficiency are beneficial as these are linked to longevity. Aerobic exercise, anaerobic exercise, food intake, environment, temperature, medications, stress, illness, metabolic disorders, medical status, menstrual status, menopause, aging process, etc can all affect our metabolic rates.

Check with your healthcare provider and/or reputable healthcare information source for additional information as needed regarding caloric expenditures, caloric intakes, metabolic rates, nutrient densities, calorie counts, etc.

WHAT ARE THE BENEFICIAL EFFECTS OF WEIGHT DISORDERS?

They can be a protective adaptation to food scarcity.

They can help in certain medical, psychological or physiological conditions.

WHAT ARE THE ADVERSE EFFECTS OF WEIGHT DISORDERS?

They can cause physical and/or physiological harm due to either acute and/or chronic effects.

They can cause severe psychological stress.

They can cause and exacerbate depression.

They can markedly affect functional status.

They adversely affect social functioning.

They can kill.

WHAT CAN CAUSE WEIGHT DISORDERS?

- Excessive food intake
- Decreased physical activity
- Metabolic disorders
- Medical disorders
- Surgical disorders
- Endocrine disorders
- HPA axis disorders
- Adipostat disorders

- Genetic disorders
- Psychological disorders
- Psychiatric disorders
- Chronic stress
- Depression
- Chronic inflammation
- Environmental causes.
- Food toxins
- Food additives
- Household chemicals
- Environmental toxins
- Metabolic disruptors
- Pollution
- Miscellaneous

GENES INVOLVED IN WEIGHT DISORDERS

- MC4R
- FTO
- DRD2
- ADRB2
- ADIPOQ
- LEPRDRD2
- Miscellaneous

Multiple discrete gene loci have also been delineated in various genetic, metabolic and weight disorders.

Genetics is thought to influence about 20% of weight disorders. In addition, intake, food, behavioral, physiologic, psychological, endocrine, HPA axis function, metabolism, etc affect about 80% of Weight Disorders. All of these factors have to be considered in entirety.

HORMONES AND WEIGHT DISORDERS

LEPTIN

- Satiety hormone
- Produced by adipose cells, enterocytes, etc
- Acts on the hypothalamus
- Inhibits hunger
- Stimulates satiety
- Gene on chromosome 7

GHRELIN

- Hunger hormone
- Produced in stomach
- Acts on the hypothalamus, nucleus acumens, anterior pituitary, etc
- Increases appetite
- Acts on the cholinergic-dopaminergic reward centers
- Gene on chromosome 3

INSULIN

- Peptide hormone controlling blood sugar levels
- Produced by beta cells in the pancreatic islets
- Acts on myocytes, liver cells, fat cells, etc
- Increases fat deposition
- Counteracts glucagon
- Reduces blood sugar levels
- Decreases lipolysis, proteolysis, etc
- Affects cognition, memory, metabolism
- Present on chromosome 11

GLUCAGON

- Peptide hormone controlling blood sugar and fatty acid levels
- Produced by alpha cells in the pancreatic islets
- Increases blood glucose levels
- Converts glycogen into glucose
- Present on chromosome 2

ADIPONECTIN

- Fat burning hormone
- Secreted from adipose tissue
- Involved in glucose regulation and fatty acid oxidation
- Acts synergistically with Leptin
- Affects insulin sensitivity
- Present on chromosome 3

CORTISOL

- Stress hormone
- Produced in the adrenal cortex
- Promotes gluconeogenesis, glycogenolysis, glycogenesis
- Decreases inflammation, reduces immune function, etc
- Controlled by ACTH from the Pituitary and CRH from Hypothalamus

ESTROGEN

- Estrone, Estradiol and Estriol are the primary sex hormones in women.
- Important in lipid and protein metabolism, sexual behavior, etc
- Important in cognition, bone and heart health, etc
- Decreases binge eating

PROGESTERONE

- Endogenous steroid and sex hormone
- Important in breast development, oocyte function, pregnancy, sexual function, etc
- Increases appetite
- Major neuromodulator and neurosteroid
- Significant brain effects and anti-inflammatory function

TESTOSTERONE

- Primary male sex hormone
- Anabolic and androgenic effects
- Significant immune system, genital system and brain effects
- Significant cardioprotective effects are seen
- No evidence of increased prostate or testicular cancer with supplementation

THYROID HORMONES

- T3, T4, T3U and TSH are commonly measured.
- T4 and T3 are produced by the follicular cells of the thyroid gland.
- Thyroid hormones regulate metabolic functions all over the body including protein, fat and carbohydrate metabolism.
- They are affected by iodine and selenium deficiencies.
- Hyperthyroidism and Hypthyroidism can cause significant changes to metabolism rates in both adults and children.
- Hypothyroidism causes neurodevelopmental disorders in the prenatal period.

CATECHOLAMINES

- These are Monoamine Neurotransmitters which are important in metabolic activities.

- The commonest ones are Epinephrine, Norepinephrine, Dopamine, Serotonin, etc.

- These play important parts in Metabolism, CNS and PNS function, Stress response, etc.

- Toxins, Additives, Obesogens, Pathologic States, Stress, etc. can affect circulating levels and function.

- They affect heart rate, blood pressure, glucose levels, weight control, alertness, nervous system activity, metabolic activity, etc.

Most metabolic, hormonal and functional loops in the human body are tightly regulated and controlled. When there is a disruption of the components in these loops, presence of toxins or disruptors, presence of injury or disruption at the cellular, subcellular, molecular levels, etc, disordered function is a common outcome resulting in pathologic function.

HPA AXIS

This is an neuroendocrine axis comprising of the Hypothalamus, Pituitary and Adrenal glands.

It regulates multiple systems and functions including Digestion, Immunity, Emotions, Metabolism, Sexuality, etc.

The hypothalamus mainly secretes Corticotropin Releasing Hormone (CRH) and Vasopressin.

The anterior pituitary mainly secretes Adrenocorticotropic Hormone (ACTH).

The adrenal cortex secretes glucocorticoids, mainly cortisol. Glucocorticoids act on mineralocorticoid and glucocorticoids receptors. Cortisol acts on the pituitary and hypothalamus in a negative feedback loop.

HPA DISRUPTORS

- Stress
- Psychological states
- Overload states
- Malnutrition
- Dystopian diets
- Infections
- Microbiome dysfunction
- BPA
- PFOA
- Environmental toxins
- Food toxins
- Food additives
- Molecular disruptors
- Medications
- Pesticides
- Insecticides
- Household Cleaners
- Additives
- Pollution
- Miscellaneous

ADIPOSTAT

The adipostat is akin to a thermostat and controls both fat mass and energy metabolism. It is present in the hypothalamus. It is closely indexed with metabolism, hormones, behaviors, environment, neurochemicals, toxic molecules, cellular disruptors, psychological states, stress, etc. and indexes the body with the neuroendocrine axes. The body has evolved this over millennia and the body in addition has a weight point around which your weight is controlled. This usually balances metabolism and prevents drastic changes from affecting your weight.

WHICH CONDITIONS CAN CAUSE WEIGHT DISORDERS?

- Obesity
- Overeating
- Malnutrition
- Diabetes Mellitus
- Hypothyroidism
- Metabolic disorders
- Nutritional disorders
- Polycystic ovarian disease
- Depression
- Cardiac disorders
- Respiratory disorders
- Vascular disorders
- CNS disorders
- Toxic disorders
- Addictive disorders
- Psychological disorders
- Psychiatric disorders
- Chronic Stress
- Depression
- Hypothalamus-Pituitary-Adrenal (HPA) axis disorders

- Neuroendocrine disruption
- Genetic disorders
- Miscellaneous

WHAT ARE THE ADVERSE CONSEQUENCES OF WEIGHT DISORDERS?

- High Blood Pressure
- Lipid disorders
- Coronary Artery Disease
- Cerebrovascular Disease
- Cardiovascular Disease
- Peripheral Vascular Disease
- Diabetes Mellitus Type II
- Pancreatic disorders
- Hepatic disorders
- Biliary disorders
- Renal disorders
- Gastrointestinal disorders
- Respiratory disorders
- Musculoskeletal disorders
- Rheumatologic disorders
- Metabolic disorders
- Endocrine disorders
- Pyschiatric disorders
- Immunologic disorders
- Obstetric disorders
- Gynecologic disorders
- Sleep disorders
- Sexual disorders

- Cancer
- Miscellaneous

HOW MANY PEOPLE ARE AFFECTED BY WEIGHT DISORDERS?

As per widely published data in the literature, Weight Disorders affect more than 250 million people in the USA. These numbers are increasingly being replicated elsewhere all over the world, upto 3 billion, sometimes with greater disease burden. More definitive data might place the population affected at a much larger proportion than is currently noted.

WHAT DO WEIGHT DISORDERS COST US?

Each year, these disorders affect millions of people and cost over $ 120 billion in compensation expenditures, lost wages and decreased productivity in the USA. There are similar or higher findings reported throughout the world with probable costs in the many hundreds of billions of dollars.

WHAT ARE THE MANAGEMENT OPTIONS FOR WEIGHT DISORDERS?

Let us look at Weight Disorders in more detail. Let us look at lifestyle and management options in detail. Let us look at the complex interplay of physical, functional and psychological limitations of people affected. We will try to understand the options available and what may become available in the future. We need to look at the discrete, local and global perspectives to get us the best strategic picture and overview. This will help us in fashioning a well thought out, implementable plan.

THE LIVING SUTRAS

We all want to live well.

Living well is a journey, not a destination. Rather than be focused on arriving at the destination, let's enjoy the journey. Let's see. Let's feel. Let's be in the moment.

Let's Live Fully!!!

It's much more fun.

How do we get there?

What are some of the ways or tracks or paths we can use in our daily lives to achieve these results.

What "Sutras" or "Paths" can we follow so we can attain our goals of good health and help prevent disease, injury and pain?

Let's examine these in detail so we can use them to plan our life, take action and live better, healthier while being pain free.

If we are using some of them now, Great!

If we are using all of them, Beautiful!!

If we want to start using some or all of them now, Fantastic!!!

It's never too late to start.

If not yet started, Start Now!!!

Think and Do.

Do not think in excess.

Do not eat in excess.

Do not sleep in excess.

Do not be too active or too lazy.

Do everything in moderation.

Do not be fixated on the past.

Do not be fixated on the future.

Be in the present.

This whole world is Maya or Illusion. Do not be anxious, Do not be afraid. Exile your fears.

Be hopeful. Be happy. Lose yourself in the ways and rhythms of the Universe.

What can we do to be healthy and stay away from health problems?

What can we do now so we do well and keep away sickness, disease & affliction in the first place?

Let's use our key sutras to enlighten us, free us from ignorance and open up spheres of wisdom, knowledge and understanding.

These "Sutras or Keys to Knowledge" will unlock the secrets to living well beautifully and preventing long term problems.

Sutra "String or Thread" refers to an aphorism or string of aphorisms that enlighten us and move us forward on our Journey of Life and Knowledge. It's all a matter of choosing our paths wisely.

What are some of the things that would help with being healthy, happy and pain free?

It would be great if we are already following them.

It's even better that we start following them now!!!

What could we do now to live better and prevent pain and suffering?

How could we be healthier?

If we think of diseases or disorders as negative health states where people are weak, painful and suffering, we can also have positive health states where we are healthy, happy and content.

Life is a Journey.

The decisions we make about what we do, how we do it will influence our current state of health and also impact health over the decades to come.

How do we get there?

What can we do?

What are our options?

If we are to choose from a set of options, what choices can we consider?

What choices work if we do choose them?

Let's look at them in more detail so we can embark on a journey of good health.

As the Eight-Fold Path in Buddhism allows us to transcend suffering, death and ignorance, let's use our Living Sutras to navigate this world which is full of Maya into a land of Pure Wellbeing, Wisdom and Happiness.

May our Journey Begin!!!

THE SUTRA OF EATING WELL

We eat to live. Sometimes, we live to eat. If we mix them both, that would be a beautiful thing to do.

Our bodies will tell us how much we need. Listen well.

If we look at eating as something fun, pleasurable and beautiful, it becomes a spiritual experience. It is not work. Take your time. Enjoy.

It matters not what we eat, it matters how we eat. Eat mindfully.

Don't hate food. It will kill you. Yousa toast, baby.

If we love our food, it will love us back.

"Aharam Aushadham" is an ancient Indian saying meaning "Food is Medicine". The foods we eat and the liquids we ingest are the single biggest things that pass through our mouth and then get used by our bodies having effects on us at the macro and micro level, just like any pharmaceutical or nutraceutical. Let us be diligent therefore about what we introduce into our bodies as they have medicinal effects.

You have traditional foods used for centuries or more in varied regions of our earth. Learn from dishes, people and traditions from all around the world. Make friends with people from different cultures and origins. Obtain recipes from cookbooks and from the internet. Try new things. Look for healthier options. Open yourself to new experiences. Cheers

Always eat beautifully.

Beautiful food.

Beautiful presentation.

All that beauty will titillate you so we can eat less.

Savor the experience.

Eat fresh, local live food.

Eat food which is full of life energy or prana.

Support local, well-made produce and products. Fresh is best as it has the most and best nutrients.

Always eat food of the highest quality. Small quantities, Highest qualities.

Always eat so you are half full. Your stomach thanks you, Pardner.

Cook in high quality surgical grade stainless or traditional pots and pans. Keep away from chemical laden or chemical eluting cookware. Go traditional and borrow tools and techniques from around the world. Enjoy the experience of generations.

Always eat a balanced diet. Eat a proper mix of different foods. Eat vegetables, lentils, fruit, nuts, meat, etc. If it looks beautiful and balanced, it's good for you.

Eat in small installments. It is better on the stomach. Digestion is easier. It makes the acids, bile and enzymes work better. You will feel healthier.

Eat like the Okinawans - Hara Hachi Bu -Eat till you are 50-80% full. Your body feels lighter and your digestion works better.

Eat slowly.

Take your time.

Smell, Feel, Taste everything.

Eat when you want to. Have a few nuts, a piece of fruit, snacks, juice, etc. These are easily digested and nutrient dense.

Eat at small intervals, every 3-4 hours. Eat during a twelve hour period. Let your gastrointestinal system take a rest for the other twelve hours.

Enjoy every morsel or bite. That is such a wonderful part of life. Slow down. Take your time. Enjoy each moment.

Drink a lot of soup, every day. Eat a lot of vegetables, some meat if you like. Chop up the vegetables, pour in lotsa water, some herbs and get them to a boil. Lots of fluid intake is good. Eating a big bowl of freshly made soup fills you up. It makes you lose a lot of weight. You can lose anywhere from 20 - 40% of your body weight doing this all the time.

Drink a lot of fresh juices. Use a good juicer. Chop up the fruits or vegetables, then its right through the juicer to process. You can use the pulp in other dishes if you would like to. Better still, pulp and eat fruits whole with the juice and fiber together, like a pureed whole. The juice gives us nutrients and vitamins. The pulp is loaded with fiber and nutrients. Use all the fruits that we can. Eat daily.

Drink lots of water. Pure H20. At least two liters per day is good for most people. Follow up with your doctor for advice on water restrictions if you have any special conditions. It allows your kidneys to work better and flush out the toxins in the body. Make it a habit and drink regularly. If you drink a lot of water in the morning, about 2 full glasses, it will help you do toodle doo. It helps to regularize bowel function and facilitate bowel movements. This can additionally help to prevent colon cancer as it keeps the intestinal tubes clean. Also, we feel lighter, healthier and more energetic.

If fresh juices or fruit are not available, drink juices without additives or preservatives. Any good store should have a decent organic additive free selection. Do not drink anything with added sugar, high fructose corn syrup and chemical additives, etc. For better products and results, pulp or make your own juice.

Have a lot of fruits and vegetables. The more variety, the better it is for us. It adds a lot of fiber. Lentils, beans, oats, unrefined grains, fruits and vegetables have a lot of fiber. That helps with weight control. It helps regulate bowel function. Aim for a wide selection. High fiber intake has been shown to decrease the incidence of colon cancer.

Eat a lot of fish. Salmon, Mackerel, Trout, Herring, Sardines, Tuna, local selections like Pomfret, Hilsa, Murrel, etc are great choices. Small, oily fish are good. Anything in your lake, pond, river or sea is great, too. Broil or grill them, they are healthier. Also, if the fish have bones, we take our time to pick them out so we eat slower and mindfully.

Eat healthy fats like Olive, Avocado, Grape, Mustard, Coconut, Peanut Oils, Butter or Ghee (clarified butter), etc. Always use in moderation.

Eat healthy. Think healthy. Be healthy.

Good products in the right quantity at the right intervals.

Healthy attitude is everything.

Eat less Flour. Eat more MultiGrains and Lentils. Eat Flour with Jack fruit added to it. Eat Flour with Lentils and Super Grains added to it.

Eat Flour with SuperEnrichers added to it. Add Spinach. Add Cauliflower. Add SuperFoods. Add Fiber. Let us do the same for all other Grains too.

Eat MultiGrains. Eat Combinations of Grains. Add SuperNutrients & SuperFoods.

Flour with Jackfruit Flour may help you with Diabetes. As will adding Fenugreek or Methi to your dishes. As will eating Munakkaya or Moringa or Drumsticks - both the fruit and leaves. Onion seeds - Kalonji - may help too. Eating certain foods may keep you healthy and prevent diseases from happening i.n the first place

If you eat Turmeric, you may be able to prevent Cancer and Alzheimer's disease. Use in all your foods and others too so you can get all the health benefits.

If you use Cinnamon regularly, you may decrease your chances of getting Alzheimer's disease. It may also help lower blood sugar levels in Diabetes.

If you eat multiple Indian spices and products including Ginger, Garlic, Garam Masala, Cumin, Coriander, etc., they may prevent or help modulate Hypertension, Heart Ailments, Cancer, Alzheimer's disease, Diabetes etc. Start researching and start using herbs and spices from many varied and rich traditions worldwide. Think and Do.

Eat slower. Take your time. The extra time will allow the satiety center in the brain to be stimulated and the hunger center to be turned off. Soup, a small appetizer, fruit juice, an aperitif and good conversation all serve this purpose.

Talk more. Have great conversations. We will be healthier. Once we talk and are more alert, we tend to choke less. Also, as we talk, we take amounts of air in which will lead to less food being eaten. It will also give us more time so our satiety center kicks in before we eat most of our food.

Eat a lot of soy and other varied bean products. These have lower bioavailability than animal proteins. Bioavailability is the percentage of protein that is used by the body. Beans have a bioavailability around 30-40 % while that of animal protein is around 80% or higher. So, we digest animal protein and pack it in more. Because vegetable proteins are less digestible, they have and add far more roughage. In addition, the bacteria in the gut work on lentils or beans, which lead to musical notes. If there are fragrances, let it all out. It is good for the intestines to decompress. The more varieties of lentils we use like black beans, mung dal, red lentils, etc., the better it is for us.

Have a lot of mucho virgin olive oil. Virgins are good. Use it on salads, in cooking and as a garnish on food. There is a lot of research out there attesting to its health benefits. Use avocado and coconut oils. Use butter and ghee. Use natural cold pressed, expeller pressed or natural process extracted oils. Stay away from chemically extracted oils. Use the residuals of oil extraction for animal feed or as minimally processed foods.

Eat vitamin and nutrient rich foods. Your body needs these for optimal functioning.

Use serotonin rich foods like sweet potatoes, oranges, figs, blueberries, pineapples, etc.

Eat dopamine enhancing foods like beans, meats, nuts, seeds, broccoli, green tea, etc.

Eat GABA enhancing foods like beans, nuts, etc.

Eat acetylcholine enhancing foods like seafood, liver, eggs, etc.

If you feel any nutritional shortfall or need supplementation, take vitamins. Use high quality, bioavailable vitamins.

Eat fermented foods like Yogurt, Lassi, Kimchi, Sauerkraut, Kefir, Miso, Injera, Tofu, Dosa, Idli, Pessarattu, Vada, etc. These are great for your metabolism and health.

Eat SuperFoods like SuperProteins, SuperFats, SuperGrains, Super-Fruits, Super Spices, SuperNuts, SuperGreens, etc. Use these as building blocks to create a greener, cleaner SUPERYOU.

Aim for a 1/3 SuperGrains to 1/3 SuperFats to 1/3 SuperGrains ratio in all your meals.

Aim for a Breakfast of 30% Lunch of 30% Dinner of 30% plus Snack of 10% of your total caloric intake through the day. Enjoy.

Vitamin C: It is used by the body to maintain itself. It aids in metabolism and also makes for stronger connective tissues. Eat citrus fruits such as oranges. mandarins, limes, etc. Eat kiwi, peppers, broccoli, strawberries, gooseberries, brussels sprouts, cantaloupe. cherries, etc.

Vitamin A: We all know lack of vitamin A causes night blindness. People who have this problem can't see well at night. It is also important in immune function. Eat carrots, spinach, kale, winter squash, sweet potatoes, etc.

Vitamin E: It is an important vitamin that is important in immune, cardiovascular and visual function. It has received a lot of press recently for its antioxidant activity. It has been shown to decrease the incidence of heart attacks. Eat avocados, almonds, sunflower, olive oil, peanuts, hazelnuts, etc.

Vitamin D: This is very important in bone health. It also regulates calcium metabolism. Being in the sun gives us a good supply. If we are deficient and need some; milk, cod liver oil, supplements, etc are good sources.

Minerals and Trace Elements: These are essential to normal function of our body and organs. Calcium, potassium, magnesium, iron, selenium, chromium, zinc and other minerals and trace elements are found in a wide range of foods including nuts, milk products, etc. Supplements are also a good source.

The Chinese believe everything in this world has a certain power including foods, drinks, extracts, life forms, organs, etc. This life force can be assimilated when we eat that life form or thing. Worms, snakes, placentas, plants, aliens, etc; you get the idea. Aim for the same.

Eat to be happy.

Eat for joy.

Eat blissfully.

Savor every morsel.

Be in the moment.

Feel every moment and experience.

Strive for balance.

Eat what you like.

Eat lots of fresh yogurt. Fresh, Unprocessed, Living. Yogurt has billions upon billions of good bacteria that are necessary for proper functioning of our intestines. This helps restock and repopulate the healthy bacteria in our microbiome. This also helps in proper immune function. It gives us a good supply of calcium and protein. Lactose intolerant individuals can ingest it too as the milk lactose is eaten up by the bacteria in yogurt. It is very easy to make and enjoy fresh yogurt every day or every few days at home. You can also have it alone or with whole-pulped fruits as a light, easily digestible snack.

Eat balanced foods.

Feel the balance of foods you eat.

Balance by food types, colors, textures and smells.

Spice up your life. Use exotic spices like Turmeric, Cumin, Coriander, Cloves, Fenugreek, Garam Masala, etc. Use from your own culture and borrow from others. All of these can help save our health; prevent diseases and other undesirable conditions like Cancer, Hypertension, Dementia, etc. It is very important to research and use well as they are very good for us all. As always, Practice Moderation.

Always grind spices fresh if you can in a mortar-pestle, hand held grinder or in a spice grinder. Buy in small quantities. Buy only the best quality. Grind when you need them. You have active ingredients and you use only as much as you need of fresh ground active spice ingredients. Store them in clean glass, stainless steel or inert containers.

Use exotic flavorings like Saffron, Cardamom, etc which have been prized since antiquity for myriad health benefits.

Use antioxidant packed spices and herbs such as Cloves, Cinnamon, Black Peppercorns, Turmeric, Oregano, Rosemary, Thyme, etc. Spice up your life. Eradicate oxidants in your body. Get younger.

The Koreans have a variety of textures and colors on the plate. Eat for color. Eat different colored veggies and fruits-red, green, white, pink, yellow, etc. Eat everything under the rainbow.

Aim for diversity.

These balance us.

Aim for Balance.

Eat for quality, not quantity.

Never stuff yourself. Stay light, lean and mindful.

Aim for fresh, natural, high quality products all the time.

Invest in good quality cookbooks. Learn from millions of healthy recipes on the web and/or knowledge repositories. Learn from friends locally. Learn from friends around the world. Share and grow.

Do shop at farmers markets. Buy fresh locally grown and harvested produce and products. Do shop at good Indian, Mexican, Asian and other exotic food stores. Buy vast amounts of quality vegetables and fruits at low prices. Avoid most processed foods like the plague. Do not buy overpriced, stale vegetables and fruits from slow moving retailers or sellers. Avoid foods that have been harvested, transported or stored for long periods of time as they have low nutrient density and freshness.

Eat foods sourced from all the continents and oceans of the world.

Eat less. Studies have shown that if we decrease our caloric intake by a third, our life span increases up to 30%. If we eat low amounts of calorie dense foods, increase soup intake, eat fruit and vegetables, we are well on our way. Fast sometimes like half a day or one full day. You will be lighter and healthier. It will reset your metabolism.

Eat low glycemic index and low glycemic load foods including vegetables like Cauliflower, Cabbage, Broccoli, Mustard Greens, Mushrooms, Okra, Beans, Spinach, Brussels sprouts, etc. Use Fruits like Apples, Oranges, Pears, Peaches, Guavas, Dragon fruit, Mango, Pineapples, etc.

Use unsweetened and additive free yogurts and cheeses.

Use a wide variety of nuts and whole grains.

Eat riced veggies like riced cauliflower, riced broccoli, other riced veggies, etc.

Have a lot of dry fruits and nuts. Pistachios, Almonds, Cashew nuts, Walnuts, Pine nuts, Brazil nuts, Flax seeds, Sunflower seeds, Melon seeds, Pumpkin seeds, Apricot Seeds, Macadamia nuts, etc are great choices. They have a lot of trace elements, minerals and vitamins. Eat a palmful a day. It will increase your life expectancy and health. Use in all your curries and chutneys. Go Nuts, Sweeties.

Let it all out. Don't hold it in. All of it. Pee regularly. Fart regularly. Crap regularly. Once we empty our wastes, we keep the cycle moving. It also reduces the amounts of feces held in the body and less toxin absorption. Fiber, Probiotics Volume, Water, Exercise all help keep our intestines and intestinal contents moving. It is all good.

Be Free, My Friend.

Eat or drink in silver or gold utensils. We can source these from India where they have been in use for centuries. Trace amounts of these metals will be dissolved in the food or drink and will be ingested by us that are good for our health. Also, it's more beautiful and we will enjoy our food more.

Make every Meal a Happy, Healthy, Joyful, Beautiful, Sensual and Magical Experience.

Use organic food as much as you can. Avoid pesticide, herbicide, chemical fertilizer, antibiotic or hormone laden foods. Grow your own herbs in your garden, apartment or house. It is great for you. It is fresh and decreases our health risks while we get quality foods. Let's make ourselves and our earth healthier and more alive.

Eat foods with less toxins, pesticides, herbicides, additives, preservatives, etc. Stay away from highly processed foods. Stay away from foods packed in plastics and harmful packaging. Use food stored in sustainable, nonreactive, smart packing materials.

Eat Chyawanprash. This was developed and used by the ancient rishis, seers and monks in India. They were on a quest for self-knowledge and truth. They would undergo great austerities and fast for weeks. To keep their body functions from shutting down, they would take the Chyawanprash to keep them healthy and prevent these problems. This is made of about 40 or so herbs and minerals mixed in honey, sometimes with gold and silver mixed in and potentiated as bhasmas. Using it regularly will keep you active, younger and healthier. Top quality ones can be sourced from India.

Eat SuperFoods, SuperFruits and SuperGrains sourced from all around the World. Use wisely and benefit from the experience of millions of people and cultures all around the world using foods like Moringa, Jackfruit, Alla Neredi Pandlu (Syzgium Cumini), Sitaphal (Custard Apple), Ber or Berries, Munjalu, Passion Fruit, Dragon Fruit, etc.

Eat SuperFoods and SuperFruits like Pomegranates, Goji Berries, Jackfruit, Maca Root, Mangoes, Acai berries, Anona, etc. Eat Munakkaya, Sorakaya, Dosakaya, Kakarikaya, Bacchala Kura, Munakkaya, Gongura, etc.

Drink tea and coffee. These contain flavonoids, which are potent antioxidants. They are important in preventing heart attacks and strokes. Drink good quality, natural products of your choice. Organic foods are even better. Do everything in moderation.

Enjoy desserts once or twice a week. Use a scoop or couple of teaspoons twice per week, mate. These are good for us.

For desserts or concentrated sweet stuff like ice creams, cakes or sugary desserts, limit you maximum intake at 1 scoop. Of this amount, do the three-tablespoon rule. Eat one, sometimes two, never more than three half or full teaspoons. STOP

LIVE. ENJOY. BE HAPPY WITH LESS.

For sweeteners, use minimal amounts of Honey, Sugar, Raw Unprocessed Brown Sugar, Mishri, Stevia, Molasses-Pomegranate-Dates,

Agave, Monk Fruit, Jaggery, Fruit Purees, Fruit Concentrates, etc. Stevia is a good sugar substitute as it sweetens food without an insulin response.

Never use or reduce your use of artificial sweeteners as they have lots of adverse health effects including cancer.

Eat ice cream one or two times a week, serving size: 1 scoop or half a scoop. A tablespoonful can be more enjoyable than a half-gallon. It is all in perception. The phospholipids and lipids found in milk products may help in amelioration of various neurologic pathologies.

Eat good, delicious high-quality chocolate. Least Processed, Most Beneficial. These are packed full of antioxidants. As always, indulge in moderation.

Go unprocessed often. Use raw, good, unprocessed foods when you can.

Eat high quality cheese. It has tremendous health benefits. Always do eat in moderation. Make fondues. Eat with meals. Eat as a snack. Try new ones all the time.

- Love your food.
- It will love you back.
- Eat to Live.
- Live to Eat.
- Long live the King and Queen.
- Meditate.
- Be Mindful.
- Be Thankful.

FOOD BASICS

Clean out your Pantry, Food Storage and Refrigerator/Freezer ASAP.

Fully examine all the foods you have.

Donate or throw out all highly processed and low nutritional value foods. Stop buying them again.

Stop shopping in the center of the store-retail setting where the processed foods are. Stop buying processed foods now!!!

Always shop on the periphery in retail settings where the fresh foods like vegetables and fruits are placed.

Go buy in farmers markets,

Go buy in exotic stores like Mexican, Indian, Asian grocery stores.

Grow your own herbs, fruits and veggies if you can. Process and can on your own. .

Stop buying unneeded items or groceries. Think smart. Eat smart. Buy only the essentials.

Do not buy much. Do not waste much. Shop smartly.

REDUCE OR ELIMINATE THESE FOODS

- Highly processed foods
- Artificial sweeteners
- Foods with trans fats
- Foods with added fats
- Foods with added sugars
- Foods with added protein
- Foods with added sugar, high fructose corn syrup, fructose, etc.
- Foods with artificial colors
- Foods with chemical preservatives
- Foods with pesticides

- Foods with herbicides
- Food with artificial coatings
- Foods with antibiotics
- Foods from toxic locales
- Foods from contaminated soils
- Foods from contaminated rivers or water bodies
- Foods which are unseasonal
- Foods from far off locations, the transport of which can degrade food quality, freshness and nutrients
- Foods with administered growth hormones
- Foods made with processed grains
- Foods with nitrates or nitrites
- Chemically extracted oils
- Foods with fillers
- Irradiated food
- Food stored for long periods
- Foods transported for weeks or months
- Foods frozen for weeks, months or years
- Cheap foods
- Unsafe foods
- Toxic or unsafe packaging of foods
- Low quality foods

EAT THESE FOODS

- Eat high quality foods
- Eat natural and organic foods
- Eat natural and organic produce
- Eat wild sourced over conventionally farmed fish
- Foods made with whole grains and whole grains

- Minimally processed foods like brown rice, cut whole oats, etc
- Ethically sourced natural or organic dairy products like milk or cheese
- Ethically sourced natural or organic meats
- Natural cold pressed or expeller extracted oils
- Use traditionally made high quality foods.

ETHICALLY SOURCED MEATS

- Range or grass fed beef
- Range or grass fed lamb
- Range or grass fed goat
- Venison
- Elk
- Bison
- Horse
- Donkey
- Guinea pig
- Wild boar
- Free range chicken
- Emu
- Ostrich
- Geese
- Ducks
- Bear
- Moose
- Antelope
- Deer
- Zebra
- Water Buffalo

- Rabbit
- Rodents
- Camel
- Reindeer
- Yak
- Alligator
- Crocodile
- Python
- Snakes
- Insects
- Lizards
- Squirrels
- Reptiles
- Hedgehog
- Porcupine
- Road Kill
- Worms
- Meats from around the world
- Vegetarian meats
- Lab grown meats
- Miscellaneous

ETHICALLY SOURCED DAIRY

- Range or grass fed cow milk
- Range or grass fed sheep milk
- Range or grass fed goat milk
- Range or grass fed donkey milk
- Range or grass fed camel milk
- Range or grass fed mare milk

- Reindeer milk
- Water buffalo milk
- Reindeer milk
- Yak milk
- Moose milk
- Cheeses made from the above
- Soy milk
- Almond milk
- Oat milk
- Rice milk
- Vegetarian milks
- Dairy products from around the world
- Miscellaneous

FISH & SEAFOOD

- Salmon
- Sturgeon
- Squid
- Bass
- Shark
- Rohu
- Murrel
- Carp
- Flounder
- Grouper
- Haddock
- Monkfish
- Shrimp
- Tuna

- Halibut
- Cod
- Herring
- Mackerel
- Dolphin
- Whale
- Lobster
- Catfish
- Clams
- Oysters
- Scallops
- Caviar
- Eels
- Sharks
- Molluscs
- Crustaceans
- Seaweeds
- Fish and seafood from around the world
- Miscellaneous
- Wild caught is always better than farmed.
- Farmed with vegetarian or sustainable feed sources is better
- Line caught is better than bulk trawling.
- Always buy sustainably sourced ethical seafood and renewable freshwater sourced aquatic foods.

GRAINS

- Wheat
- Buckwheat
- Millets, a wide variety from India, China, Africa and worldwide

- Oats
- Teff
- Brown Rice
- Quinoa
- Non GMO Corn
- Sorghum
- Barley
- Rye
- Kamut
- Pumpernickel
- Chia
- Amaranth
- Spelt
- Miscellaneous

LENTILS

- Chickpeas
- Peas
- Moong Dal
- Toor Dal
- Masoor Dal
- Black Dal
- Chana Dal
- Red Lentils
- Kidney Beans
- Black Beans
- Pinto Beans
- Lima Beans
- Soybeans

- Pigeon peas
- Fava beans-Foul medemmes
- Peanuts
- Miscellaneous

VEGETABLES

- Arugula
- Seaweed
- Spinach
- Kale
- Mustard greens
- Swiss chard
- Cauliflower
- Cabbage
- Brussels sprouts
- Eggplant
- Cucumbers
- Munakkaya-Moringa
- Kandagadda
- Kohl Rabi
- Gongura
- Bacchala Kura
- Gongura
- Potatoes
- Capsicum
- Peppers
- Mushrooms
- Pumpkins
- Squash

- Carrot
- Sweet Potato
- Turnip
- Beet root
- Onions
- Garlic
- Ginger
- Beerakaya
- Potlakaya
- Sorakaya or Opo
- Eggplant
- Methi
- Karve Paku
- Cilantro or Kothimir
- Mint
- Parsley
- Dill
- Chives
- Muli
- Radish
- Miscellaneous

FRUITS

- Mango
- Mangosteen
- Rambutan
- Sapota
- Cherries
- Plums

- Pears
- Peaches
- Alla Neredi Pandlu
- Sita Phal
- Falsa
- Currants
- Guava
- Grapes
- Apples
- Tomatoes
- Raspberry
- Blackberry
- Blueberry
- Acai berry
- Strawberry
- Bilberry
- Lingonberry
- Cloudberry
- Raspberry
- Cranberry
- Ber
- Kumquat
- Watermelon
- Honeydew
- Tarbooz
- Pineapple
- Papaya
- Pomegranate or Anar
- Apricots

- Oranges
- Grapefruits
- Tangerines
- Lemons
- Limes
- Jackfruit
- Munjalu
- Cashew
- Kiwifruit
- Lychees
- Passion Fruit
- Dragon Fruit
- Dates
- Star Fruit
- Miscellaneous

SNACKS

- Traditional Snacks
- Vegetables
- Fruits
- Sunni Undalu with Jaggery
- Palli Undalu with Jaggery
- Cashew Chikki with Jaggery
- Kachori
- Dhokla
- Pav Bhaji
- Pani Puri
- Chaat
- Fresh yogurt

- Sev
- Bhujia
- Egg Puff
- Meat Puff
- Masala Chickpeas
- Masala Phalli
- Sattu Pindi
- Appalu
- Garelu
- Sakinalu
- Arishelu
- Cottage cheese
- Kue
- Gavvalu
- Mini Sliders
- Bread with olive tapenade
- Pickled olives
- Kebabs
- Soups
- Salads
- Sandwiches
- Cheeses
- Multigrain breads
- Chole Bhature
- Puri with mango
- Bread-omelet
- Dappi
- Boiled eggs
- Omelets

- Popcorn
- Pretzels
- Bagels
- Edamame
- Seaweed
- Granola bars
- Jerky
- Sausage
- Meats
- Tapas
- Pork Rinds
- Smoothie
- Egg puffs
- Cookies
- Cakes
- Pastries
- Miscellaneous

NUTS

- Almonds
- Pistachios
- Walnuts
- Pecans
- Hazelnuts
- Pili nut
- Pine nut
- Candle nut
- Malabar Chestnut
- Mogongo nut

- Yeheb nut
- Brazil nut
- Macadamia
- Cashew nuts
- Coconuts
- Miscellaneous

FERMENTED FOODS

- Yogurt
- Sauerkraut
- Kefir
- Kumis
- Natto
- Shubat
- Smetana
- Skyr
- Vietnamese fish sauce
- Miso
- Soju
- Kombucha
- Injera or Ethiopian fermented wraps
- Kimchi
- Fermented chilies
- Lassi
- Shrikhand
- Dosa
- Vada
- Idli
- Various pickled foods from Koreas, India, China etc

- Mead
- Miscellaneous

CHEESES

- Gouda
- Edam
- Brie
- Asiago
- Branzi
- Gruyere
- Emmental
- Chhurpi
- Ema Datshi
- Mozzarella
- Mascarpone
- Cheddar
- Parmigiano Reggiano
- Queso Fresco
- Gorgonzola
- Stilton
- Wensleydale
- Ricotta
- Pecorino Romano
- Provolone
- Camembert
- Havarti
- Bavarian Blue Cheese
- Cambozola
- Edelpilzkase

- Hirtenkase
- Weiblacker
- Munster
- Roquefort
- Valencay
- Provolone
- Bergader Almkase
- Reblochon
- Feta
- Fine Goat Milk Cheeses
- Fine Sheep Milk Cheeses
- Fine Donkey Milk Cheeses
- Fine Camel Milk Cheeses
- Fine Exotic Cheeses
- Miscellaneous

SPICES AND CONDIMENTS

- Cumin
- Coriander
- Jeera
- Black pepper
- Red pepper
- Allspice
- Garam Masala
- Bay Leaves
- Cloves
- Nutmeg
- Pasupu or Turmeric
- Ginger

- Garlic
- Tamarind
- Sumac
- Saffron
- Cinnamon
- Paprika
- Mace
- Asafoetida
- Miscellaneous

OILS

- Ghee
- Butter
- Coconut oil
- Extra virgin olive oil
- Lard
- Tallow
- Mustard oil
- Peanut oil
- Palm oil
- Rice bran oil
- Safflower oil
- Sunflower oil
- Canola oil
- Saffola oil
- Soybean oil
- Corn oil
- Linseed oil
- Hemp oil

- Avocado oil
- Sesame seed oil
- Almond oil
- Castor oil
- Grape seed oil
- Walnut oil
- Miscellaneous

FAMOUS FOODS

- Biryani
- Pulau
- Kebabs
- Nasi Goreng
- Idli Sambar
- Wada Sambar
- Rasam
- Pappu Charu
- Ulava Charu
- Vangibath
- Appam
- Ragi Mudde
- Rava Dosa with Chutneys
- Masala Dosa
- Kachori
- Haleem
- Hareez
- Nihari
- Steak
- Chicken or Beef Broccoli

- Baked Salmon
- Pizza
- Goulash
- Blood sausage
- Pork chops
- Pork knuckle
- Borscht
- Pelmeni
- Fried-Grilled-Barbecued Chicken, Fish, Beef, Mutton, Goat meats etc
- Mutton curries
- Chicken curries
- Fish curries
- Prawn curries
- Seafood curries
- Vegetarian curries
- Spanakopita
- Grilled octopus
- Khichdi
- Dal Roti
- Dal Chawal
- Dum Pukht
- Pork Knuckle
- German Style Sausages
- Fried Fish and Seafood
- Fried Noodles with Seafood
- Pho
- Baked or Fried Pomfret
- Lobster with Butter
- Meatloaf

- Dalpuri
- Chengdu Hot Pot
- Wiener schnitzel
- Chapala Pulusu
- Royyala Curry
- Daddojanamu
- Pulihora
- Smoked Salmon
- Hawaiian Luau
- Fusion foods
- Samosas
- Chaat
- Pani Puri
- Vadapau
- Rogan Josh
- Grilled vegetables
- Brazilian rice with beans
- Pad Thai
- Grilled noodles with seafood
- Pho
- Spinach omelets
- Veggie omelets
- Dal Makhani
- Dal Bhati Churma
- Gatte Ki Sabzi
- Kadhi
- Keema
- Sarson Ka Saag
- Chole Bhatura

- Puri
- Peking Duck
- Spaghetti with meatballs
- Momo
- Tandoor
- Mongolian stir fry
- Chicken Manchurian
- Chow Mein
- Raabdi
- Bhagara Baingan
- Kheema
- Dim Sum
- Barbecued Ribs
- Nasi Lemak
- Congee
- Satay
- Curry Mee
- Lapsha
- Oliviet
- Varenniki
- Baba Ghanoush
- Hummus
- Kibbeh
- Kitcha fit-fit
- Ceviche
- Empanadas
- Burritos
- Seafood Chowder
- Crab cakes

- Gumbo
- Burgers
- Lasagna
- Polenta
- Bisque
- Foie Gras
- Bouillabaisse
- Salade Lyonnaise
- Fiskesuppe
- Foraged Salads
- Miscellaneous

FAMOUS DESSERTS

- Double Ka Meetha
- Gulab Jamun
- Payasam
- Kissel
- Laddu
- Baklava
- Rasagula
- Petha
- Shrikhand
- Malpua
- Halwai
- Rabri
- Modak
- Kalakhand
- Trifle pudding
- Jalebi

- Apricot pudding
- Umm Ali
- Gajar ka halwa
- Kaddu ka halwa
- Beetroot ka halwa
- Rose petals halwa
- Badam katli
- Kaju katli
- Egg pudding
- Kulfi
- Crepes
- Gelato
- Ice creams
- Ras Malai
- Dry fruit barfi
- Cookies
- Cakes
- Walnuts with honey
- Apfelstrudel
- Sachertorte
- Moon Cake
- Miscellaneous

BEVERAGES

- Water
- Carbonated Water
- Milk
- Tea
- Coffee

- Hot chocolate
- Lemonade
- Iced Tea
- Root Beer
- Milk Shake
- Indian Chai
- Sherbet
- Cider
- Beer
- Whiskey
- Rum
- Vodka
- Gin
- Wine
- Cognac
- Armagnac
- Brandy
- Port
- Floral teas
- Fruit teas
- Coconut water
- Indian Style Almond milk
- Beverages from around the world
- Miscellaneous

UTENSILS

- Pure silver cutlery and utensils
- Pure gold cutlery and utensils
- Coated gold cutlery and utensils

- Coated silver cutlery and utensils
- Pure stainless steel cutlery and utensils
- Bone China
- Porcelain
- Specialized alloy cutlery and utensils
- Stone cutlery and utensils
- Jade cutlery and utensils
- Miscellaneous

Eat well

THE SUTRA OF DRINKING WELL

Drink alcohol. It is good for you. It will help you relax and decrease your stress. Alcohol is a stimulant and a depressant depending on the amounts and timing of use. Use everything in moderation.

Drink a lot of water. It's the nectar of life. Drink at least 8 ounces of water at least 8 times a day for about 2 liters or about half a gallon a day for most people. More is always better as per your needs and activity and you decide what's best for you. For any special disease states or conditions, ask your doctor.

Drink lots of fresh or bottled juices, bottled without any additives or preservatives. Do not drink juices with added sugar, high fructose corn syrup, artificial and/or chemical additives.

Drink coconut nectar, straight from the fruit if you can. Otherwise, use a well bottled or packed product. Try to use unprocessed or minimally processed products. Stick to nature that has mastered and refined processes over thousands of years.

When you get up in the morning, drink at least two full glasses or 500 ml of water on an empty stomach. It will rebalance your stomach after an overnight fast, help you go poo poo and rehydrate your body while cleaning out the tinkly tinkly pipes.

Do store water in a silver-ragi-steel-gold jug and/or an Indian ragi chambhu or flask, especially overnight. The silver utensil leeches small amounts of ions and oxidation products into the water which is very healthy for our bodies. If you can afford gold, get one and use it daily.

Carry water in clean stainless-steel flasks or vacuum flasks or glass bottles. Stop using plastic bottles which are terrible for the water and the environment. Plastic bottles leach a myriad of chemicals into the water inside, none of which is good for you. Use non-reactive glass or steel surfaces. Save your money, save your health and save our environment. Always reuse.

Check your water in a quality lab. Always make sure you have access to the best quality water. Research all options well. Do not blindly believe in brands or charlatans. Invest in specialized water purification systems as needed. Your body and health is worth a lot more.

Drink coffee or tea, as you wish. Feel the flavonoids. Use freshly made natural ones using just in time processes. Use your judgement. Drink well, prosper.

Add mint or sacred basil (Indian Tulasi) to your water. Drink hot or warm water. Different Chinese or Indian philosophies theorize that these warm or hot fluids are better for you and your metabolism.

Make and drink fresh tea. Instead of just drinking one variety all the time, aim for variety. Aim for flavors. Choose herbicide and pesticide free organic teas. Try floral teas. Try herbal teas. Try rare ones from around the world.

Avoid bottled teas like the plague. They are usually full of sugar, preservatives and dated tea products. Drink fresh.

Make and drink fresh coffee. Try different ones from around the world. Go organic. Pay and ship directly from producers. Try to source most products locally if you can. Cut out sugar, syrups, artificial flavors and preservatives as they massively add to our sugar and fat intake while being deleterious to our health.

Cut out conventionally grown ones made with pesticides, herbicides and toxic chemicals. A lot of these disrupt your metabolism and your weight. Choose pure products.

Use a juicer, make fresh juice. Squeeze the flesh, baby. It's relaxing, we get juice and we still can use the flesh. We can blend the pulp into desserts or food dishes. Use whole fruits. We can also use it to make vodka or ethanol.

Try to have pulped whole fruit juice or purees and/or homogenized fruit either with your meal and/or as a snack. A glass or two is good for you. You will eat less. The satiety center is satiated. You will also lose weight.

Drink water flavored with real fruit and herbs. Lot of these have vitamins and minerals that are good for you. Drink Fresh and Drink Pure.

Being well hydrated at all times is imperative for your health and well-being. Your skin glows. You look and feel healthy. Everything works well.

Drink high quality dairy products. Milk. Almond Milk - Indian Style. Cardamom Milk, Soy Milks, etc are all good. Hooray, Me Love Dairy Moo. Use fresh local products.

Drink fermented foods like Indian Lassi, Kefir, etc. These are great for your intestinal and general health.

Drink clean, good, high quality alcohol. Less than 2 drinks a day and upto 8 drinks per week is a good guide to living well. Drink only as much as you like or enjoy.

Drink beer like the Germans. It's great for your stomach, your happiness and your life. It will help flush you out, keep your kidneys and pee pee pipes clean and nice. Have fun. Enjoy responsibly with friends. Drink fresh. Drink local.

Draught beer is fresh and tasty. Draught is always better than bottled. Fresh bottled is better than aged or stored ones. Drink German, Belgian, Czech, etc. beers with a lot of tradition. Drink seasonal beers such as summer, autumn, Oktoberfest, winter ones, special occasion, etc.

Drink local fresh or bottled beer from around the world. There are a lot of fantastic beer varieties from all around the world. Try something new.

If you don't use alcohol, use nonalcoholic beers. You can use boiled barley water too.

Cognac, brandy, whiskey, vodka, beer, whatever is good and whatever shakes yore boat, Das Kapitan.

Drink to experience. Smell. See. Savor. Enjoy the full experience.

Do not drink to get drunk, unless you really want to. Make sure you are around someone you know. So, when you pass out, you have someone to carry or drag you home. Better to wind up safe than sorry.

Drink socially. Drink with friends, strangers, anyone. Soon, the strangers become less strange or become friends.

Buy someone a drink. It's good for your health. Plus, if it's the right sex, you might just score.

Do not drink and drive. Sleep over or better still, sleep with the barmaid or barman, wherever your taste runs.

Engage people in conversation. You just might learn something new. Drink, Live, Learn.

Eat small tidbits while you drink. Eensy meensy bitesy. Eat kebabs, nuts, finger foods, etc. while you drink. You won't get drunk that fast. You also don't become hypoglycemic. It makes drinking more fun. Remember, it's all about enjoying the experience.

If you drink a little alcohol, it is a stimulant. You speak like Aristotle. You feel great, are confident and aroused.

Do not ingest more than 2 drinks per day. Better stick to 8 drinks or less per week.

If you drink a lot, you slobber, drool and feel like a stuck pig. Also, the little general goes on vacation and doesn't work. Get the idea. Moderation is always a great idea.

Too much alcohol can hurt you. People get Cirrhosis, Cancer, Dementia and a host of other conditions and diseases. Moderation is the mother of all things.

Try spritzers, diluted spirits with aerated-carbonated products, fruit juices, etc.

Try traditional or local tipples like Neera, Kallu or Coconut water. Very healthy and good for the gastrointestinal system too as they tend to flush you out. Experiment. Enjoy. Use.

Enjoy drinking. Tipple, but do not topple.

Drink beautifully. Enjoy the experience. No other way, Baby.

Quality, not Quantity is Primo. Experience a wide range of tastes.

Laugh a lot. Laugh alone. Laugh with friends. Tell jokes. Watch funny movies or clips. Laugh together and the Universe laughs with you.

Make someone happy. Make anyone happy. Cheers.

May the force be with you.

Enjoy, Compadres

FINE BEERS

- Heineken
- Peroni
- Hefeweizen
- Singha
- Brahma
- Asahi
- Kingfisher
- Haywards
- Kolsch
- Marzen
- Pilsener
- Pilsner Urquell
- Gambrinus
- Primus
- Bock
- Chinmay
- Paulaner
- Carlsberg
- Hoegaarden
- Stout
- Guinness
- Ale
- Stella Artois

* Lindemans
* Modelo Especial
* Negro Modelo
* Corona
* Pabst
* Tsingtao
* Molson
* Labatt
* Kirin
* Sapporo
* Hite
* Miscellaneous

FINE WHISKEYS

* Johnnie Walker Black Label
* Johnnie Walker Blue Label
* Ballantyne
* Bell
* Chivas Regal
* Caol Ila
* Laphroaig
* Lagavulin
* Port Dundas
* Aberlour
* Black Bull
* Glen Scotia
* Glenmorganrie
* Macallan
* Auchentoshan

- Aultmore
- Balvenie
- Talisker
- Oban
- Peter Scot
- Midleton
- Hibiki
- Dalmore
- Fine Single Malts
- Fine Blended Malts
- Miscellaneous

FINE COGNACS

- Remy Martin, VSOP or XO
- Hennessy
- Hine
- Martell
- Tesseron
- Laubade
- Delamain
- Courvoisier
- Camus
- Miscellaneous

FINE VODKAS

- Grey Goose
- Chopin
- Imperial

- Absolut
- Tito
- Hortitsa
- Wyborowa
- Miscellaneous

FINE RUMS

- Diplomat XO
- Old Monk
- McDowell
- Bacardi
- Ole Nassau
- Ron Mulata
- Dictador
- Dos Maderas
- El Pasador de Oro
- Miscellaneous

FINE WINES

Red Wines

- Chateau Cissac
- Chateau Tronquoy-Lalonde
- Flor de Pingus
- Cote de Brouilly
- Second Voyage
- Arte Ante
- Riojas
- Beaujolais

- Pinot Noirs
- Malbecs
- Syrahs
- Merlots
- Tempranillos
- Miscellaneous
- White Wines
- Chardonnay
- Sauvignon
- Riesling
- Muscat
- Chablis
- Miscellaneous

Rose Wines

- I Capitelli
- Le Reveur
- Bertrand Cote Des Roses Rose
- Chateau Miraval Cotes De Provence Rose
- Franzia Sunset Blush
- Miscellaneous

Champagne & Sparkling Wines

- Veuve Clicquot
- Moet & Chandon
- Mailly Brut Reserve Grand Cru
- Prosecco
- Rondel Brut Cava
- Miscellaneous

Plum Wines

- Hoshi
- Takara
- Fu-Ki
- Gekkeikan
- Kikkoman
- Miscellaneous

Fruit Wines

- Elderberry wine
- Pomegranate wine
- Pineapple wine
- Dandelion wine
- Rose hip wine
- Red currant wine
- White currant wine
- Orange wine
- Prune wine
- Lychee wine
- Cherry wine
- Blueberry wine
- Mulberry wine
- Seaberry wine
- Raspberry wine
- Miscellaneous

Mead

- Sky River Mead Sweet
- Dansk Mjod Viking Blod Mead

- Bunratty Mead
- Lindisfarne Mead
- Chaucer's Mead
- Miscellaneous

Ice Wine

- Inniskillin
- Moet & Chandon Ice Imperial
- Wagner Riesling
- S Sohne
- Freixenet Ice Cuvee
- Miscellaneous

Rice Wines

- Sake
- Rihaku Wandering Poet Sake
- Hakutsuru Sayuri Junmai Nigori
- Gekkeikan Black & Gold
- Mura Mura Mountain Sake
- Tozai Snow Maiden
- Miscellaneous

Sato

- Mijiu
- Beopju
- Dansul
- Miscellaneous

- Miscellaneous Fine Spirits

FINE TEAS

- Darjeeling
- Ootacamund (Ooty)
- Assam
- Floral
- Herbal
- White
- Yellow
- Green
- Oolong
- Black
- Fermented Tea
- Puerh
- Masala
- Chai
- Jasmine
- Exotic Teas
- Miscellaneous

FINE COFFEES

- Ethiopian
- Brazilian
- Colombian
- Chikkamagaluru
- Malabar
- Nilgiri
- Madras Coffee
- Civet Dung Coffee

- Elephant Dung Coffee
- Exotic Coffees
- Miscellaneous

FINE PUREED FRUIT & WHOLE FRUIT JUICES

- Mango
- Sapota
- Cherries
- Plums
- Pears
- Peaches
- Alla Neredi Pandlu
- Sita Phal
- Falsa
- Guava
- Grapes
- Apple
- Tomatoes
- Raspberry
- Blackberry
- Blueberry
- Acai berry
- Ber
- Watermelon
- Honeydew
- Tarbooz
- Pineapple
- Papaya

- Pomegranate or Anar
- Apricots
- Oranges
- Grapefruit
- Tangerines
- Lemons and Limes
- Jackfruit
- Munjalu
- Cashew fruit
- Dates
- Miscellaneous

MISCELLANEOUS DRINKS

- Bobo
- Unsweetened Carbonated Soda
- Badam or Almond Milk
- Saffron Milk
- Apple Cider
- Non Alcoholic Beer
- Soy Milk
- Almond Milk
- Cashew Milk
- Rice Milk
- Coconut Milk
- Coconut Water
- Hot Chocolate
- Neera
- Kallu

- Ragi Malt
- Kombucha
- Miscellaneous

Eat Well
Drink Well

THE SUTRA OF LOVE, HAPPINESS AND SPIRITUALITY

It is amazing how much love there can be between people who have met on this journey we call life.

Love is an act of our Will.

Love is a Phenomenon.

Love is a Feeling.

It can be personal or impersonal. It can be unidimensional or multi-dimensional. It may or may not involve sexual desires.

It is a multidimensional, multisensory experience. It involves, people, animals, things, ideas, et al.

We can choose to Love. Or Not. It's our choice.

It is so easy to choose to love. All it takes is intention and the ball is in motion.

Love

It is an electromagnetic net or force field that envelops all lifeforms and the entire universe in its being.

The Universal Integrator.

What a thing to live with.

What a thing to live without.

We can love people, ideas, objects, souls, the universe, etc. We can love anything and everything. It is not about anything; it is about us. It is a state of mind. It is a state of being.

It is an empire of love.

An empire that is without boundaries or barriers.

An empire that is without classes or creeds.

An empire that is ever bountiful and self-sustaining.

An empire that is lighter than a feather but spans the entire universe.

What if we said to ourselves?

I love rain.

I love sunshine.

I love snow.

I love storms.

I love myself.

I love my neighbor.

I love my neighbor's wife. Just kidding, but you know what I mean!

Actually, I love to love everything.

Love can make everything alive.

Love can heal.

Love can create love.

Love is balance.

Love is harmony.

Send love outwards. Draw love inwards. Love Love. Love.

Good things happen to good people.

Bad things happen to good people.

Anything can happen to anyone.

But, if we love ourselves and others, we can always make anything work for us.

In Tibetan and Jewish cultures, there are traditions where you let go of negativity and bad thoughts. We will ourselves to let go. It is in essence a way of exorcising these so we can fill up with positivity, hope and love. It is essentially moving away from darkness to light.

Our body is a Temple. Let's take care of it well in multiple dimensions.

Physically.

Emotionally.

Spiritually.

Different faiths all agree on eating and drinking moderately, taking care of our bodies, health and environments in addition to focusing on our mental and spiritual needs. Being at peace and equilibrium with ourselves and the universe are core tenets of health and happiness.

But sometimes, this may not be enough.

As in the Indian tradition, we can look at being involved with good and positive people - Sat Sangh – a meeting of the good. People sit down and sit down with a good book or a good philosopher or a precept and discuss things in detail. It is a way to get connected. It's a way of getting involved. It stimulates us. It creates enthusiasm. It leads to an increase in consciousness.

Go to your Temple. Go to your Church, Synagogue or Mosque. Go to a secular temple like a park or a forest or a lake. Engage with people and the community. Volunteer. Feed or share with the less fortunate. Stop clinging or hoarding. Start sharing.

Share your belongings. We come into the world with nothing, We leave with nothing. So why hang onto ephemeral things? Stop Collecting. Start Sharing. Own very less. Feed your neighbors. Feed the hungry. Respect all beings.

Surround yourself with good people. Perform good karma. You will collect the fruits. Start today. Why wait?

This creative engagement makes our hearts lighter and mind ablaze with knowledge. Let your mind be free and boundary less.

Open your mind.

Welcome the world in.

Get busy in your home and street and neighborhood and city and country and the world. See what you like. Explore. Engage.

We do not need to have everything going for us to be happy.

Things can happen to us, good or bad.

It is our response to these events that determines whether we can and will be happy. Getting over adversity is ennobling for our spirit.

We want to be happy.

We need to be happy.

We can be happy, not only when good things happen to us but also when bad things happen. It is a choice.

We can choose to be happy. Happiness is a state of mind. Happiness is a choice.

Happiness, I believe, is being plugged into the love that is all around us. Love is harmony. It is connecting with all the energy and love of the Universe.

Let it all go.

The clinging.

The fear.

The greed.

The avarice.

The longing.

Let it all hang out.

See it for what it is.

Let It All Go!!!

Stop running after money or material objects like a dog. Better, Be the Dog and be happy with nothing. All we really need are food, love and belonging. Give away all your possessions. Own very less. Share everything.

Get a dog, cat or other pet. They will help decrease your blood pressure and reduce your risk of heart attack and stroke by over 30%.

Pet owners are found to be more connected, more loving and less stressed. The less stress, the healthier you are and the longer you live. They increase serotonin levels while decreasing cortisol levels.

Pet owners get more exercise, are more active and more social which is all great for our health.

Most pets are selfless and take in the world around with a sense of wonder, pleasure and gratitude. These are great qualities that we can inculcate in ourselves so we respond to the universe at an elemental level. This frees us to reach higher states and respond harmoniously to the energies and rhythms of the universe.

Janmamu Satyame - Birth is Certain!

Mrithuyu Satyame - Death is Certain!

These are the only two true realities. Ignore false realities, fears and desires.

We come with nothing: We leave with nothing.

Illuminate your mind.

Dispel your illusions.

Let go of empty desires and tribulations in this temporary impermanent world.

This material world with all its temporary desires, fears and longings is all Maya.

It is all a Dream.

It is all an Illusion.

Pierce the Veil!

Watch the Universal Cosmic Dance.

Be in control.

Be controlless.

What exactly is control?

Who has control?

Is there ever control?

Lose the illusion of control!

Help people who are less fortunate around you. Giving will make you better, happier and more involved. Purposeful activity is the best antidote to worry.

Sex, togetherness and connectedness are great for us. They help improve our mood, stress levels and happiness. Sex helps increase release of dopamine, serotonin, oxytocin, etc. Sex balances out the sex hormones in our bodies. Sex indexes our neuroendocrine axis and balances our energy fields.

Sex and Love connect us to the Eternal, Mystical, and Cosmic Forces underlying the Universe. We get to connect blissfully with God and/ or the Universe!!!

We can cultivate love.

We can cultivate happiness.

Happiness is harmony.

Love is harmony.

Life is harmony.

May you be at peace with the world, my friends!

LOVE

- Friends
- Family
- Pets
- Charitable Activities
- Social Activities
- Work
- Religious Activities
- Spiritual Activities
- Knowledge
- Awareness
- Sex
- Love
- Miscellaneous

HAPPINESS

- Spiritual Activities
- Sex
- Love
- Knowledge
- Awareness

- Friends
- Family
- Pets
- Charitable Activities
- Social Activities
- Work
- Religious Activities
- Miscellaneous

JEWELLERY & ART

- Pure gold necklaces and jewellery
- Pure silver necklaces and jewellery
- Pure platinum necklaces and jewellery
- Diamonds
- Rubies
- Emeralds
- Corals
- Pearls
- Paintings
- Sculptures
- Precious Stones and Minerals
- Fine Jewellery & Objects
- Fine Art
- Miscellaneous

RELIGIONS

- Hinduism
- Islam
- Christianity

- Buddhism
- Zoroastrianism
- Jainism
- Sikhism
- Jewish
- Animism
- Scientology
- Bahai
- Folk Religions
- Miscellaneous

SPIRITUALITY

- Zen
- Taoism
- Confucianism
- Kabbala
- Vedanta
- Sufi Movement
- Bhakti Movement
- Yoga
- Animism
- Voodoo
- Miscellaneous

Eat Well
Drink Well
Love Well & Be Happy

THE SUTRA OF SLEEPING WELL

Sleep is a restorative.

The body heals itself while we sleep. It uses surplus energy that we use during activity to repair itself. We wake up after a refreshing sleep feeling like a million bucks.

Sleep can be serene and restful. Very often, such is the case. If not, let's get it back to normal levels.

Sleep can be interrupted by physical or psychological distress. Minimize these if you can to the greatest extent possible.

Develop a sleep routine. Routines are good.

Create a calming relaxing atmosphere.

Take a shower. Once or twice a day, unless you live in the Sahara desert and see water once every few weeks. In which case, take a pitcher of water and you can sponge yourselves with a wet cloth or towel. Wipe yourselves fully daily or every few days. These rubs will have a relaxing, massaging effect. Reuse the water to sustain a few trees or plants. Do drip irrigation. Drip some water for multiple plants or trees. Sustain and Invigorate Life. Waste not, Want not. Recycle the water. Conservation is the best policy in life.

Swim in the sea. Use a pool. If you are near the sea, swim in the sea. Swimming is good for us all. Cleanliness is good for our bodies and our souls.

Get a massage, from your partner, neighbor or willing provider. Do your own massage with hands or devices. Pay for it if that's what makes them tickle you. Give a massage, Get a massage. Free is Best. Enjoy.

Exercise daily. It will work off all the excess energy. It normalizes body rhythms. It makes you breathe better. It's good for your heart. It also relaxes you.

Try to use a Sauna and/or Jacuzzi every day or every few days. It will make you sweat and massaged. It will rev up your metabolism. It will increase your endogenous endorphins. It makes you feel better and sleep better.

Breathe deeply. Become one with the Universe.

Practice meditation. Be mindful, earthling.

Get a drink, enjoy it. It will ease your passage into that slumberous wonderland.

Do sex and lotsa boom boom. Every day, if you can! It's great for your body, mind and psyche. It is a wonderful connecting exercise. It's relaxing, healthy and puts you in a nice state of mind. It helps you sleep like a baby.

Sleep balances our regular sleep wake cycles. It helps balance our hormone levels so we are healthier and happier. It is very important to have homeostasis.

No Televisions or Electronic Devices in your sleep area. Period. If you have too many Televisions, consider donating them to the less fortunate in your community. All you need is one good one, preferably in the living room which is a common shared area.

If you have too many televisions or electrical-electronic devices, it ups the electromagnetic force fields all around you. As we are all essentially electromagnetic beings, we are intimately affected by all the radiation fields around us. Abnormal force fields may cause diseases and result in abnormal functioning of organ systems. Decrease these and be more intimately connected to nature.

DeTox regularly from chemical, electrical, electromagnetic and/or other pollution states regularly.

Throw a comforter and pillows on the ground. Try sleeping on the floor. Get in touch with the earth. Notice the effects of its magnetic fields. Try some new sex and sleeping positions on the floor. Hey, Kitty, Kitty.

Try Tatami Mats. Try Indian Soppa Mats, Japanese Tatami mats or similar ones elsewhere. Try Dhurries. Try comforters or leather rugs. Try wooden floors. Try concrete floors. Try the living ground. You need contact for all your body parts to be grounded, centered, connected, flexible and able. Walk barefoot as much as you can..

Try not to think of sleep. Don't think too much. Let it whisk you away in its arms on its own.

Hold someone or something. Touch is good.

Do not use excessive stimulants or depressants.

Use medication only as needed. If you need it, use it.

If you can't sleep, do something till you feel sleepy. Try new positions, areas, actions, etc.

Take a short nap if you can, short is sweet. It is healthier, makes you more productive and is good for your heart. A short nap can decrease your risk of heart attacks by up to 60%. Siestas such as in Spain, India, etc are great for health, wealth and longevity.

Try sleeping on your lawn. Sleep on your porch. Sleep on the beach. Sleep wherever you can. Always listen to your natural rhythms.

Chill out. Don't worry too much. Inhale. Exhale.

Develop sleep rituals. Develop what works best for you. There is no one size fits all.

Do not let it get too warm or too cold. Extremes are bad. They cause problems going to sleep or wake you up in the middle of the night. They may be bad for your organ systems too including the respiratory system.

Meditate. Do Breathing Yoga. Visualize beautiful mindscapes.

Sleep like a Dog or Cat.

Just surrender to sleep and relaxation.

Don't fight it. Don't overthink it. Just do.

Be happy. Try to be if you are not. It will work out eventually.

Laugh a lot. Try to be thankful for all the good you have or will have.

Enjoy sex or relaxing in your bed. Enjoy your floor. Enjoy your car. Enjoy in Nature. Enjoy all over this beautiful world. Have fun everywhere!

Get lucky. Do it Daily, Weekly or Monthly.

Enjoy, My Friends.

Listen to beautiful music. Music calms your senses. It equalizes brain waves so you wake up refreshed. Music will calm your rhythms. You can cure diseases or conditions with the right soundscapes and actions. Experiment & discover using creations from all over the world. Find what you like.

If you can do so, get solid wood beds shipped from India. Use traditional natural cotton mattresses. Get a charpoy with jute netting, Use natural cotton and wool coverings.

Sleep naked or clothed. See what works best for you. Enjoy!

Try Indian Bhajans. These are beautiful, melodious chants. Try local or exotic music. Try singing yourself. Do whatever relaxes calms and soothes you.

Look at beautiful art, objects and/or people. Whatever tickles you is good. It will put you in a good mood. It uplifts your mental state and consciousness.

If you have sleep apnea, narcolepsy, restless legs syndrome, respiratory, neurologic, cardiopulmonary, musculoskeletal or multisystem disorders, etc.; please see your doctor or healthcare professional for care to help fix these problems.

Visualize beauty and peace. Do daily and as much as you can. Use all avenues of your body, mind and consciousness.

Help someone. It will help you build good karma. Find what you can do for others. It will help you as much as them. Giving is the best way of receiving blessings. Get blessings every day from yourself, your family & friends and all around the Universe.

Lie in bed. Think. Let your thoughts go. Empty your mind. Mediate. Focus on your breath. Do simple asanas. Let it all go. Breathe.

Be Happy.

Be Relaxed.

Be Thankful.

Be Blissful.

HERBS-SUPPLEMENTS FOR SLEEP

- Lavender
- Valerian
- Lemon
- Thyme
- Chamomile
- Ashwahgandha
- Melatonin
- Miscellaneous

FOODS PROMOTING SLEEP

- Milk with Cookies
- Nuts with Honey
- Desserts
- Honey
- Fruits
- Rice Pudding
- Almond Milk
- Rice with Meat Curries
- Rice with Yogurt
- Small Sandwiches
- Tapas
- Snacks
- Yogurt
- Lassi
- Kefir
- Alcohol
- Miscellaneous

MUSIC FOR SLEEP

- Evening Ragas
- Evening Bhajans
- Instrumental
- Classical
- Relaxing Soundscapes
- Lullabies from around the World
- Miscellaneous

BEDS & MATTRESSES

- Charpoy
- Fine Solid Wood Indian Beds
- Fine Indian Natural Sleeping Gear
- Hammocks
- Leather Furniture
- Metal Furniture
- Water Beds
- Air Inflatable Beds
- Hospital Beds
- Comforter on Floor
- Floor
- Fine Carpets
- Fine Mattresses
- Fine Beds
- Miscellaneous

SLEEP DISRUPTORS

- Stimulants
- Drugs of Abuse
- Caffeine
- Alcohol
- Noise Pollution
- Light Pollution
- Noxious Smells
- Unhealthy Surroundings
- Unsafe Surroundings
- Extremes of Temperature
- Cardiopulmonary Disorders
- Respiratory Disorders
- Musculoskeletal Disorders
- Toxic Psychological States
- Toxic Mental States
- Sleep Disorders
- Miscellaneous

ACTIVITIES PROMOTING SLEEP

- Exercise
- Sex
- Mild to Moderate Drinking
- Unwinding routine at end of day
- No TV in bedroom
- No Electronic Devices in bedroom
- No loud noises or music
- Non confrontational conversations

- No caffeine or stimulants after 4 PM
- Shower
- Massage
- Sleep rituals
- Prayer
- Light snack
- Proper sleepwear
- Proper temperature
- Essential oils or fragrances
- Mosquito nets or specialized devices as needed
- Meditation
- Miscellaneous

Eat Well
Drink Well
Love Well & Be Happy
Sleep Well

THE SUTRA OF BREATHING WELL AND MINDFULNESS

Breathe well and deeply.

It's Frei, Frei and Frei.

Inhale fully.

Exhale fully.

Do over and over. It's great for you.

Breath is Life. The more you breathe, the more you live. You live better, smarter and longer.

Check out Pranayama or Breathing Yoga. Learn Pranayama in Yoga, "Prana" referring to life or breath and "Ayama" for practice or routine. It will clean your body and mind. Learn from a good teacher or online. Go slowly and smartly so you can learn and do the right way.

Qigong from Tai chi is similar and great too. Use what you like.

Drink in the oxygen from the sea of air all around us.

Inhale and extract oxygen.

Exhale and remove carbon dioxide.

Do over and over.

Do a full inhalation so your chest fills up.

Do a full exhalation so your chest empties.

Keep going, over and over.

Focus on your breath. It will equalize you with the rhythms of the universe.

Enjoy breathing.

Focus.

DeFocus.

Make it effortless. Play with all these rhythms of life and nature.

Take time to breathe. Connect with the rhythms of the universe.

Learn as needed or desired from a good teacher, as needed. Do it all in moderation.

Learn to breathe well. Many techniques are available. All of them are pretty good. Do whatever works best with you.

Do not take yourself seriously. Breathe. Let it all go.

Relax. Actively Destress. Just Breathe.

Take in the world around you. Appreciate its beauty. Become one with it.

Make sure you are in an area with not too many allergens or toxins. Take all steps to mitigate all these well if so needed. Let's all get involved so we always have access to clean air resources in all our communities worldwide.

Clean Earth.

Clean Air.

Clean You.

Invest in proper air filtration systems. Help clean up the air and environment in your neighborhood. Do shramdan or free shared activities. Start something good. Be fully involved. It only takes one to change the world or start the process.

Use Electrics or Hybrids. Use clean public transport. Do ridesharing. Do crowdsourced rides. Walk. Bicycle. Use cycle rickshaws. Use horses, donkeys or oxen driven transport. Travel less. Work remotely if you can. Telecommute as much as you can. Work less and work smart. Share more. Use less fossil fuels. Use more biofuels. Care for and renew your and our world.

If you have allergies, avoid triggers. Go consult all the appropriate specialists. Do whatever helps you get better. Use your lungs and airways better. Always get the best diagnostics, imaging and therapeutic options.

If you can, change your environment so it's the best for you. Let us lobby and have your governments clean up around us.

Life is the most precious gift for all of us, The Best Ever.

Exercise well. You will appreciate what breathing does for you. Excellent health and performance benefits will materialize and potentiate.

Exercise by yourself. Exercise with friends. Exercise with groups.

Swim well. It will help you breathe well. As swimming is an excellent mix of strokes, rhythm and breathing, it's one of the best exercises known to man.

Hold your breath underwater. Swim underwater. It will increase your cardiovascular endurance. Increase your cardio respiratory endurance progressively in stages. The more you do, the better you get. Also, it makes you appreciate breathing a whole lot more.

If you have medical conditions that hamper your lung or heart functions, please consult your doctor for the best recommendations. Most conditions may be remediable with proper medical care.

If you have cardiovascular, respiratory or other conditions, consult your doctors immediately. Get all diagnostics and care as needed. Consider a Cardio Pulmonary Rehabilitation program. If it's a neuromuscular issue, have it fully investigated and managed by your doctors and healthcare teams. If you need specialized equipment, so be it. Get what you need.

Breathe 100% oxygen sometimes. It helps us to take ourselves to a higher level.

Exercise daily.

Get out in Nature.

Breathe well, Deeply and Gratefully.

Use hyperbaric chambers. You are in a pressurized chamber with 100% oxygen. This will make you look younger and better. You can also get up to 20 times the amount of oxygen that is normally present in your body. Let us clean everything out. Let's potentiate our functioning. Oxygen is sexy, Baby.

Learn to breathe well and deeply.

Let go.

Let it all go.

Meditate.

Connect with the Universe.

MINDFULNESS

Be mindful.

Be in the moment.

Be there fully.

Open your mind.

Illuminate your mind.

Unleash your mind.

May the Energy of your Mind Fuse and Dance with the Energy of the Universe.

It is all a state of mind.

It is a state of being.

Be in the moment.

The mind is fickle. But it can be controlled. Imagine a chariot with horses. Imagine a chariot without horses. Get the idea. Control.

Good things happen.

Bad things happen.

Anything can happen.

What is not important are the stresses, insults or trauma. It's what our response to it is.

Life is full of pain and joy. Learn to appreciate both mindfully.

Aim for balance.

Let the mind be a friend, not a foe.

The mind can be either our greatest friend or our greatest foe.

Only we decide which way it goes.

It can either be with us or against us.

Better choose wisely.

Straddle and span the opposites.

Look beyond both illusions to the truth.

Breathe.

Attain a state of desirelessness.

Do not desire pleasure.

Do not desire pain.

Let go of desire.

A state of desirelessness is Nirvana-Heaven.

Heaven and Hell are both around us as we are suspended in the infinity of space.

We can choose.

Choice is life.

Choose well.

We enter into the world with nothing.

We leave this world with nothing.

Why then be attached to unnecessary belongings, connections or fears in this ephemeral world?

Let Everything Go.

Concentrate on the Real.

Do not focus on the Unreal.

Be Free.

Chant Mantras.

Chant Prayers.

Sing.

Lose yourself in the rhythms of the Universe.

Let go of the fruit of action.

Concentrate on action alone.

"Nishkama Karma" - Ceaseless action without desire. Act smartly.

Meditate.

Open up your mind.

Open up your consciousness.

Open up to the infinite rhythms and expanse of the Universe.

Connect.

Let Go.

Be Blissful.

Think.

Solve.

Enjoy.

We can use the power of positive thinking, mindfulness and intention to make ourselves better.

Think of pain that affects you as an unneeded or unwelcome guest.

You definitely do not appreciate or want the pain.

Let the pain go.

Let the pain disappear.

Relax your mind.

Relax the painful area or areas in your body.

Feel the pain, tightness, hurt, negative energies and stress slipping away from you.

Bid the pain, tightness, restrictions and suffering goodbye.

Empty Your Mind.

Meditate.

Fill yourself, your body and mind with relaxation.

Fill yourself with gratitude.

Fill yourself with peace.

Repeat as often as you like.

Repeat hourly.

Repeat every half hour or hour of your life.

Repeat Daily. Every Day of your life

Repeat Weekly.

Repeat Monthly.

Repeat Yearly.

Repeat all the time.

Be free of pain and suffering.

Fill yourself with light, gratitude and happiness.

BREATHING

- Pranayama
- Zen
- Pulmonary Exercises
- Spirometry
- Pulmonary Rehabilitation
- Cardiac Rehabilitation
- Thoracic Breathing
- Abdominal Breathing
- Qigong
- Miscellaneous

MINDFULNESS TRAINING

- Ashtanga Yoga
- Vinyasa Yoga
- Hatha Yoga
- Bikram Yoga
- Laya Yoga
- Kundalini Yoga
- Tantric Yoga
- Pranayama
- Buddhist Yoga
- Jain Yoga
- Tai Chi
- Aikido
- Zen
- Martial Arts
- Mindfulness exercises
- Miscellaneous

Eat Well
Drink Well
Love Well & Be Happy
Sleep Well
Breathe Well & Be Mindful

THE SUTRA OF EXERCISING WELL

Exercise improves activity, balance, movement, develops strength and endurance.

It improves all of our functional systems, especially the cardiovascular, respiratory and musculoskeletal ones.

It improves our immunity and helps us stay young and fit. It helps in the antiaging process.

Aerobic exercise uses large muscle groups and helps increase oxygen usage. Examples are running, rowing, tennis, etc.

Anaerobic exercise increases muscle mass, strength, bone density. Examples are weight training, sprinting, high intensity interval training, etc.

Flexibility exercises increase range of motion, stretching and agility.

We have extensive evidence showing the beneficial effects of exercise on the Cardiovascular, Respiratory, Skeletal, Immune, Central and Peripheral Nervous Systems. It tones our biochemical and hormonal processes. It affects sleep in marked ways.

Exercise every day. From 5-10 minutes to 30-45 minutes or more, whatever tickles you.

You will be healthier, happier and wealthier.

Help someone with their life. You will break a sweat.

Laugh a lot. Daily. Laughing is exercise too and burns a lot of calories. It helps blunt the effects of daily stress.

Walk everywhere.

Walk anywhere.

Walk all the time.

Walking is a great exercise. It conditions your cardiovascular, pulmonary and nervous systems. You breathe better. You feel better. You are connected.

Do walking meditation. The cadence or rhythm, consistency and mindfulness of walking induce a meditative mode which helps enhance our mind body connections. Right foot forward. Left foot forward. Repeat.

Try to exercise at least an hour a day. More or less than that works too. Anything is better than nothing at all.

Try Tai Chi. Work with a coach and learn well. Do in groups. It is great for flexibility, strength, balance and is good for all age ranges. The benefits are invaluable for older people but the benefits can be enjoyed through all our lifetime.

Tai chi is an ancient Chinese discipline. It promotes self reliance, is meditative and has tremendous health benefits. It promotes longevity. It is based on balancing our life forces, yin and yang.

Qigong is valuable for its focus on coordinated movement, breath and awareness. It trains and promotes the life force while inducing balance.

Yoga is a blend of physical, mental and spiritual practices to train both the body and mind. It has been in practice since around the 6th century BC. It aims to unite us with the divine. It helps your strength, flexibility, mental equanimity, general health and mindfulness. It tones and strengthens multiple organ systems including the cardiovascular, musculoskeletal and nervous systems.

Though yoga is thought to be mainly about asanas, body postures, breathing or movements, it is much more. The main components of yoga are the following:

Karma Yoga: The Yoga of Action

Bhakti Yoga: The Yoga of Devotion.

Jnana Yoga: The Yoga of Realization or Knowledge.

The ultimate goal of Yoga is to help us fuse our Individual Consciousness with Universal Consciousness.

Zen focuses on realizing our true inner nature and focuses on meditation, breathing and self control. It cherishes generosity, sharing, morality, energy, contemplation or meditation and wisdom.

Try different types of martial arts like Krav Maga, Aikido, Taekwondo, Karate, Muay Thai, Jiu Jitsu, etc. Try disciplines from all around the world. Do Individually. Do in Tandem. Do in Combination. All are good for flexibility, strength, conditioning, self-defense, balance etc. Trained citizens are self reliant and make a better society.

Exercise with people if you can. If not, Exercise on your own. Exercise in your house. Exercise in a park. Exercise in your house. Exercise in a Gym. Do what you like. Always be free.

Do exercise with your body. Do exercise with your mind. Do exercise with your consciousness. It's all helpful. It's all important.

Sex is the best exercise, stabilizer and physical conditioner. The Best Ever.

Make love, either daily, weekly, monthly or yearly. Whatever suits you is best. It's a great workout and stimulant. It will condition and connect you well with your partner. Enjoy the give and take. Sweet

Play with yourself. Very helpful, dynamic and improves your mind body connection. Make your own stress-free state and boost your endorphins

Play with your pet. Go for walks. Pets are a great way to enjoy companionship and exercise while benefitting both immensely.

Breathe. Slow in, Slow out, Continue. Repeat. Delicious

Stretch. It is great for suppleness, resiliency and smart living.

Make a connection. Connect with people, lifeforms and stuff around you.

Volunteer to help someone. That is great exercise too. It has lots of mutual benefits.

Work is exercise too. Be fully involved. Enjoy your work. Work is not just for Profit. Work is Love.

Play Kabaddi. Try Baithaks in Hanuman Vyamshala, Try Wrestling. Try Gilli Dandul. Try sports, exercise regimens and martial arts from around the world.

Do High Intensity Interval Training, Metabolic Circuit Training. Resistance Training, Stretching, Aerobic Conditioning, Anaerobic Workouts, Isometrics, Isotonics, Competitive Running, Weights Training,

Yoga-Hatha Yoga, Bikram Yoga, Pranayama, Static Training, Flexibility Training, Plyometrics, Pilates, Balance Training, Martial Arts, Swimming, etc.

Use all of these modalities smartly. None is mutually exclusive.

Always work with your Physician, Athletic Trainers, Coaches, Teachers, etc. so you get the best benefits safely and perform smartly while avoiding injuries during exercise.

High Intensity Interval Training uses a warm up period, short high intensity workouts at near maximal intensity alternating with moderate intensity workouts followed by a cool down period. Examples include Running, Rowing, Stair climbing, etc.

Resistance training uses weight or resistance at 40-80% of maximum capacity at multiple repetitions. Examples include Weight training, Circuit training, Isometrics, etc

Metabolic circuit training combines interval training with resistance training to get the best benefits. Examples include Circuit training, Combo training, Paired set training, etc.

While Exercising, aim for Consistency, Variety, Progression, Smart Workouts, Moderation, Skilling, etc.

If you are standing or moving around versus sitting, your mortality rates decrease around 50% or more. Be active. Whether you walk 1000 or 10,000 steps per day, it's all good. You decrease risk of disease and death. You feel better. You burn calories..You feel alive.

Feed the hungry. It is great exercise for individuals and groups. You are feeding god. It keeps you alert and active. Go help in soup kitchen or do on your own. The concept of "Langar" in Sikh Gurudwaras is a great tradition of feeding everyone who attends and also the poor, homeless and deprived. It is a wonderful idea and needs to be more widely done all over the world in all religious institutions. When we give freely in joy, we receive massively. Hoard less. Share more. Receive more. Wow.

Do gardening. It has distinct physical and psychological effects. It helps us relate to nature. The interaction is health and rewarding. It makes us enjoy the beauty of nature and bonds us to our surroundings. Develop a passion and pursue it. You will also get either produce or pleasure. Enjoy!!!

Do volunteer work in neighborhoods by cleaning up. You help others. You help yourself. It is time to spend time in our neighborhoods while helping others and ourselves.

Go help a neighbor. In any way you can. What you receive is multiples of what you give. Complete the Circle.

Be Active.

Be Energetic.

Share!

Give of yourself freely and without hesitation.

You will prosper well.

Interact Mindfully.

Connect with the Universe.

Get off yore ass, babykins.

AEROBIC EXERCISE

- Elliptical Trainer
- Indoor Rowing
- Bicycling

- Walking
- Running
- Skating
- Skiing
- Skipping or Jumping Rope
- Skateboarding
- Swimming
- Martial Arts
- Aerobics
- Circuit Training
- Tennis
- Squash
- Basketball
- Soccer
- Football
- Dancing
- Marathons
- Cutting Firewood
- Miscellaneous

ANAEROBIC EXERCISE

- High Intensity Interval Training-Running, Rowing, Cycling
- Sprinting
- Weight Training
- Functional Training
- Interval Training
- Eccentric Training
- High Intensity Sports
- Miscellaneous

FLEXIBILITY TRAINING

- Ashtanga Yoga
- Vinyasa Yoga
- Hatha Yoga
- Bikram Yoga
- Laya Yoga
- Kundalini Yoga
- Tantric Yoga
- Pranayama
- Buddhist Yoga
- Jain Yoga
- Tai Chi
- Aikido
- Zen
- Martial Arts
- Miscellaneous

MARTIAL ARTS

- Karate
- Judo
- Aikido
- Jiu Jitsu
- Krav Maga
- Sumo
- Muay Thai
- Kalaripayattu
- Wrestling
- Dangal

- Kung Fu
- Taekwondo
- Fencing
- Archery
- Kickboxing
- Ninjitsu
- Miscellaneous

COMBAT TRAINING

- Boot Camp
- Basic Forces Training
- Special Forces Training
- Kalaripayattu
- Kung Fu
- Karate
- Swordplay
- Martial Arts
- Miscellaneous

Eat Well
Drink Well
Love Well & Be Happy
Sleep Well
Breathe Well & Be Mindful
Exercise Well

THE SUTRA OF WORKING WELL AND AGING WELL

Work is God.

Work is Life.

Work is Love.

Work is whatever we do when we are not sleeping or inactive.

Work may not always be fun but we can make it so. Try to do what aligns with your inclination, your talent, your abilities, your aims, your goals and what you expect to engineer in the results of your actions.

Work and resultant activity are great for our cardiovascular, respiratory and brain health. It's good to be active.

Movement is life. Moving around reduces cardiovascular mortality.

Work is not always about money. It can be whatever fulfils you. Do what excites you. Do what you love. Don't like what you do, Do something else.

Sometimes, people are injured, hurt or disabled and we as a society need to help them contribute to society and humanity to the best of their abilities.

Sometimes, work has become devoid of meaning or utility. Just the rote action of working is not helpful or meaningful. We need to challenge our assumptions and meaningfully explore all realistic and smart options.

One great way we need to look at is Universal Basic Income, Living Wage or Living Income where we give every person a basic sum of money. In addition to this, they can add to it by getting a job, doing business or contributing in their best way possible to our neighborhoods societies. This way, we help all people by contributing to their life while minimizing waste and inefficiencies in government and societal spending. We minimize crime, poverty, wars, etc.

When we spend only on common defense & essential services while eliminating a lot of waste in government spending, people get what is really their money. The whole world and all of our peoples benefit. A lot of waste, inefficiency and unnecessary spending is eliminated. No need to start unnecessary wars. No need to jail large sections of society. No need to keep people poor and deprived. No need to starve whole sections of society. No need to endanger the health of sections of society. Everyone is free to spend their own money their way. They may choose to work or not work. It will unleash a burst of creativity, higher order living and allows every person to do what is essentially meaningful for them.

There is always the concept of "Nishkama Karma-Ceaseless action without desire". More than work, let's empower people to be their best and contribute in any way they can so we have a better, just and smarter society.

Be Humble.

Help others.

Share.

Once we work, we appreciate leisure more. Contrasts are great.

We Work.

We Act.

We Age.

We DeAge.

Live well.

Age well.

We live well. We age well. It is the Circle of Life.

Taking care of ourselves better will help this journey. This is a process.

Have a partner through life. Have a family. If you like being by yourself, be happy. Have friends and neighbors. Be involved in community.

Love yourself.

Love others.

Age gracefully.

Loving well.

Sharing well.

Living meaningfully.

Living thoughtfully.

Living beautifully.

Pay off your debts. Cut down loans. Live simply. Live happily with less. Get rid of your worries and your burdens. Give unneeded possessions away to the less fortunate or those in need..

Make money. Spend less. Save everything you can. Be happy.

Use high end technologies such as advanced diagnostics and therapeutics including Disc Decompression, Hyperbaric Medicine, Genomics, Stem Cell Therapeutics, Natural Therapeutics, Precision Medicine, Remote Surgery, Robotic Surgery, Nutrition & Pharmacology, etc to help ourselves.

We can keep ourselves vibrant, happy and loved at any age. It is up to us to take care of ourselves and our health.

Make any and all assistive technologies available.

Make family, human or animal helpers available as needed.

Anticipate problems.

Diagnose problems.

Fix problems.

We will soon need to invest tremendous amounts of money in taking care of the elderly. We are young, we grow old and we all need care. Better invest in ourselves and our societies. Let us all pair or partner up and take care of each other.

Age is just a number.

Ignore it fully.

Be active.

Engage in your neighborhood, your place of worship and society. Help mentor young people. It's great to keep our brains and bodies active. Be respectful and live a good life. Help those around you and you help yourself.

You never need too much; Give away your belongings. Feed a neighbor. Care for a neighbor. Clothe a neighbor. The more you give away, the richer you get. Cheers.

Money and possessions are artificial, manmade constructs. Never confuse Maya or Illusion with Reality. Let us liberate ourselves and move smartly into the future.

WORKING

- House Work
- Manual Work
- Professional Work
- Trade Work
- Construction Work
- Armed Forces Work
- Services Work
- Volunteer Work
- Technical Work
- Miscellaneous

AGING

- Individual Responsibilities
- Societal Responsibilities
- Retirement
- Full Time Work
- Part Time Work
- Volunteer Work
- Living Facilities
- Living Provisions
- Medical Care

- Surgical Care
- End of life Care
- National Imperatives
- Miscellaneous

LEISURE

- Golf
- Tennis
- Rowing
- Yachting
- Pool-Billiards
- Chess
- Go
- Shatranj
- Pacchese
- Ping Pong
- Squash
- Racquetball
- Baseball
- Basketball
- Cricket
- Croquet
- Gilli Dandul
- Dangal
- Badminton
- Pickle ball
- Soccer
- Football
- Walking

- Hiking
- Mountain climbing
- Fishing
- Skiing
- Scuba diving
- Vacationing
- Travel
- Gastronomy
- Hobbies
- Miscellaneous

Eat Well
Drink Well
Love Well & Be Happy
Sleep Well
Breathe Well & Be Mindful
Exercise Well
Work Well & Age Well

THE SUTRA OF LE SEXE BOMBA

Sex is important.

Sex is not love.

Sex is an accompaniment to love.

Sex is life.

Love makes sex better.

Sex is the best exercise. Ever.

Have lotsa sex. Every single day. All day. once daily. twice daily. once weekly, once monthly or, once a year. Whatever works for you is good Pardner.

Good for your heart, Good for your life. Good for your brain. Good for your happiness. Good for your consciousness. Good for world peace.

Do traditional, untraditional and novel sex. Try new things as often as you can. Use everything.

Love and treasure your partner, lover or whoever.

Be Grateful.

Be Thankful.

Be Curious.

Get massages, regular or sexual ones. It's all good.

Show and express your appreciation and love daily.

Sex is a window into our souls. It's a window into our universe. Start traveling.

Life is a cycle.

Love others and Love yourself.

It all comes back to you.

Feed the cycle of Love.

Having sex is exercise, actually the best exercise ever invented. It's great for your body, your brain, your heart etc. You get your heart and brain active and get fantastic endorphins. You aren't as loony and you will stave off dementia.

The connectedness is great.

Relax and Enjoy.

Having sex is equivalent to running a few miles each time you engage in it. It promotes cardiovascular, respiratory and nervous system health. Sex can reduce blood pressure, decrease heart attacks, decrease strokes while making us calmer, happier and smarter. Sex balances our energy fields.

Think of sex as bonding. Think of sex as movement. Think of sex as exercise. Think of sex as dance. Think of sex as work. Think of sex as play. Whatever you think of it, it's great.

Do sex often. Get frisky. Be active. Be stimulated. Do licky licky. Do humpy pumpy. Keep the pipes and chakras clean and in top fettle.

It is great for your body.

It is great for your health and mind.

It is great for your spirit too.

If you like your partner or lover, that is great.

If not, that is great.

Get a new one or ones. Better be happy than unhappy.

When you have great sex, you are awash in pineal gland secretions like DMT-the bliss hormone. This is the same hormone seen in the higher enlightened states of spiritual gurus. Talk of sex and spirituality connecting us to the source.

Know Yourself.

Know God.

Know the Universe.

Orgasms are blissful experiences which give us a taste of and connect us to the divine within and all around us.

Control Yourself.

Control the Universe.

Think less.

Do more.

Be open.

If you like humans, Great!.

If you like Dolls, Mannequins, Sex Robots, Humanoids or Cyborgs, the Power is with You!!

If you are better alone, beautiful. You have found yourself. Play with yourself. You have all you need, your body, mind and brain. Self pleasuring is a very smart, personal, solo flight into bliss. It is a great workout too just like actual sex. It is great both for your body and brain. It is all very motivational and inspiring.

There are no fixed constants in life. See what you like and do it. Discover your own path.

Sex opens up new levels of consciousness and can open up chakras or gateways to our inner universe. As we elevate our consciousness, we truly see that our inner universe and our universes are connected seamlessly. When we truly see, we see that they are one and the same.

When we awaken our chakras and open gateways into our consciousness, we are connecting with the divine within us. We then embody the power of the universe in ourselves.

Sex is a transcendental experience. It allows us to connect with our physical, our metaphysical and spiritual planes.

Sex is sacred. We all need to celebrate the divine feminine and divine masculine in us. This helps in our spiritual development and in ascending various planes of consciousness. Tantra can be very liberating on many planes.

Be open. See what you like. Ask for it. Take your time. Release preconceptions, tension and resentments. Surrender to the pleasure. Let it wash all over your body and mind. Find your sacred core and release. Explore.

You can help prevent dementia, depression and lots of other serious medical conditions. Get moving. Get screwing. Get living.

If you have had a heart attack, pneumonia, stroke, amputation or other serious illness, get right back to sex after taking your doctor's advice. It's a very useful and rehabilitative modality, just like any exercise prescription.

If you have an erection problem, physical or mental issues holding you back, investigate fully and fix all problems with your doctors and healthcare teams. This may include, sex specialists, surgeons, urologists, physiatrists, obstetricians and gynecologists, neurologists, therapists, psychologists, psychiatrists, etc.

For any concerns or problems of any kind including performance issues, phobias, psychological problems, consult your dedicated doctors and healthcare teams. .

Ask for help.

Get helped.

Ask and you shall receive.

Sleep naked.

Walk naked.

Dance naked.

Love your body.

Love yourself.

Love your mind.

Go naked on the beach. If you like, join a commune or community. Enjoy your body.

Enjoy being naked.

Spend lots of naked time in your house or domain.

Touch yourself and massage yourself daily. It makes us feel better and keeps us healthy. It makes us know ourselves better.

Self knowledge is very life giving and heals us.

It works great for both pussy and dick. It is your choice, sweeties.

Sweet.

Use your head.

It is a very usable object.

It is better to leave inanimate objects and animals alone, unless approached and/or agreeable.

Love someone.

Love something.

Connect.

Get with the rhythm, baby.

Love everyone and everything.

Be happy and make others happy.

Celebrate.

Sex is a liberating, life giving and expansile force. It connects us to ourselves and the universe. Sex and orgasms induce bliss and release hormones, chemicals and neurotransmitters which takes us to higher planes of being.

Time to take flight, Sweeties.

Enjoy Sex.

Celebrate Sex.

Proselytize or Evangelize Sex.

Get to know yourself.

Get to know God.

It's yore life, Pardner.

The only one you got.

Get it moving.

Get it on.

All the time.

Rejoice.

SEX

- Traditional Sex
- Lesbian Sex
- Oral Sex
- Gay Sex
- Bisexual Sex
- Transsexual Sex
- Electronic Sex
- Virtual Sex
- Robotic Sex
- Android Sex

- Tantric Sex
- Kinky Sex
- Interspecies Sex
- Extraterrestrial Sex
- Miscellaneous

Eat Well
Drink Well
Love Well & Be Happy
Sleep Well
Breathe Well & Be Mindful
Exercise Well
Work Well & Age Well
Do Sex Well

THE SUTRA OF SINGING, MUSIC & DANCING WELL

Sing.

Try to sing all the time. It will put you in a good mood. It will decrease your heart rate. It will equalize your breaths. It will develop your lungs.

Sing in the shower.

Sing whenever, whatever, however, wherever and with whomever.

Listen to glorious music.

Explore different genres.

Listen to what you like.

Lose yourself in music.

Connect with the rhythms in nature.

Sound is one of the basic, elemental components of life. It's an electromagnetic force like light.

It's all energy. Our bodies respond to and incorporate good vibrations from the universe.

Watch operas and concerts. Watch dance recitals. Watch enjoyable events.

It's good for their bottom line.

It's good for your bottom line.

It's good for your life.

You don't need to be good. You don't need to be a professional. You don't need an audience. You don't need rewards. Just do for yourself. Enjoy.

Once you sing, you move. You exercise your face, throat and larynx. You exercise your lungs and heart. You exercise your body, arms and legs. You exercise your brain. You exercise your joints. With movement, you enhance both your cardiopulmonary and musculoskeletal endurance. You reset your proprioception and improve your balance.

Listen to music from around the world.

Listen to local music.

It's all good for you.

Sing with friends.

Sing in your place of worship, whatever, wherever, however, whenever and with whomever.

Make music too. Use your voice; Use an instrument, small or large.

Take music lessons. Learn. It's great for your body, mind and brain.

We are all made of electromagnetic forces. Music is too. We respond at an elemental level to the music all around us.

Music is life.

Music heals.

Go choose an instrument.

Start playing.

Start learning.

Dance, Dance, Dance.

Shake a leg, shake something. Just do it.

Move baby, like your life depended on it.

Movement is Life.

Dancing develops rhythm. It sure burns a lot of calories too.

You range your joints. You stretch your muscles. You improve your balance. You better your cardiovascular endurance. You breathe better. You move better. Your senses are more acute. Your brain is more active. What's not to like!

Life is like dancing. You don't want to be stepping on your partner's toes all the time but also you don't want to dance on the other side of the room. That is, unless you really want it to be kinky.

Try out belly dancing, pole dancing, erotic dancing, etc. It will exercise your body, mind and spirit. It allows you to free up your mind and allows you to feel and enjoy the pleasure. Do on a schedule or unscheduled. Do with a partner or friend or in groups. Join a class or do it at the gym. Enjoy the wild side.

A sexy dance might get you lucky. Try the Tango or anything where you are physically and emotionally close together.

Hola Senorita or Senor!!!

Join a dance club.

Go to a nightclub

Dance in your homes.

Dance by yourself.

Dance with your family.

Dance with your friends.

Life is rhythm.

Get with the rhythm.

Dance in the shower.

Dance in the living room.

Dance with people.

Dance in crowds.

Shake something.

Dance with your partner

Dance with your pet.

Lose yourself in the rhythms and the movements of the universe.

Connect!

Move!

Surrender!

Enjoy yourself.

SINGING

- Individual
- Group
- Contemporary
- Classical
- Bhajans
- Choir
- Religious
- Spiritual
- Opera
- Mantras
- Yodeling
- Crooning
- Humming
- Whistling
- Miscellaneous

MUSIC

- Contemporary
- Classical
- Pop
- Country
- Blues
- Jazz
- Opera
- Choir
- Bhajans
- Mantras

- Religious
- Spiritual
- Yodeling
- Piano
- Organ
- Guitar
- Ukulele
- Drums
- Cymbals
- Veena
- Sitar
- Sarod
- Tabla
- Flute
- Accordion
- Clarinet
- Cello
- Violin
- Mandolin
- Trumpet
- Bassoon
- Miscellaneous

WESTERN CLASSICAL MUSIC

- Bach
- Chopin
- Beethoven
- Brahms
- Mendelssohn

- Rachmaninoff
- Tchaikovsky
- Gregorian chant
- Folk melodies
- Haydn
- Handel
- Salieri
- Shostakovich
- Strauss
- Stravinsky
- Vivaldi
- Wagner
- Instrumental
- Vocal
- Opera
- Bocelli
- Pavarotti
- Miscellaneous

INDIAN CLASSICAL MUSIC

- Hindustani
- Carnatic
- Qawwali
- Instrumental
- Vocal
- Pandit Bhimsen Joshi
- Pandit Jasraj
- Mohammad Rafi
- Lata Mangeshkar

- Bombay Sisters
- M.S. Subbalaxmi
- Allah Jilai Bai
- Kumar Vaasu
- Kishore Kumar
- Maharajapuram Santhanam
- Dr Balamuralikrishna
- Anuradha Paudwal
- Ghantasala
- Hariprasad Chaurasia
- Nusrat Fateh Ali Khan
- S Janaki
- Tansen
- Kabir
- Purandara Dasa
- Tyagaraja
- Ustad Shaujat Hussain Khan
- Ustad Vilayat Khan
- Jagjit & Chitra Singh
- Zakir Hussain
- Abida Parveen
- Sabri Brothers
- Kumar Gandharva
- M.S. Rama Rao
- Tyagaraja
- Purandara Dasa
- Gundecha Brothers
- S. P. Balasubramaniam
- Yesudas

- AR Rahman
- Miscellaneous

WORLD MUSIC

- Tibetan
- French
- Caribbean
- Island
- Tribal
- African
- Latin
- Fusion
- Miscellaneous

DANCING

- Classical
- Contemporary
- Modern
- Ballroom
- Tango
- Odissi
- Bharatanatyam
- Kathakali
- Ballet
- Disco
- Samba
- Salsa
- Waltz

- Bhangra
- Circle
- Tap
- Miscellaneous

Eat Well
Drink Well
Love Well & Be Happy
Sleep Well
Breathe Well & Be Mindful
Exercise Well
Work Well & Age Well
Do Sex Well
Sing, Do Music & Dance Well

THE SUTRA OF LOVE AND BEING

Love yourself.

Love thy neighbor.

Love thy neighbor's wife, just kidding. Maybe!!!

Love a pet.

Love something.

Love people at work. That is, unless they are already plotting to kill you. Ha Ha!

Love people everywhere.

Love people who love you.

Love people who hate you. See, if you get close, you can slip in the knife faster.

Love people you want to love.

Love people who you love to hate.

Love everyone. It makes you a better person.

Love everything.

Lose yourself in love.

Feel the love all around you.

GOOD RELATIONSHIPS

Try to relate. If you can't, try really really hard.

Relate to everyone. Relate to your friends, family, acquaintances, strangers, etc. Relate at work, at home, at the gym, etc. See what works. If you can, that's good. If you can't, that's good. Chill.

Try to do things with others, Socialize. Slow down. Be less impatient and driven. Be more tolerant. Good for your physical and mental health.

Do things for others and help others. Help yourself.

Relate to everything including your environment, neighborhood, society, world, universe, etc.

Relationships significantly impact our health.

Relate to the Universe.

Sometimes, it's easier than relating to that crazy demented neighbor of yours.

COMPASSION

The most compassionate are the most noble.

Have compassion for yourself, your family, your neighbor, your neighborhood, your society, your country, your world.

Forgive others.

Forgive yourselves.

Become free.

SPIRITUALITY

Mahatma Gandhi.

Mother Teresa.

Marie Curie.

Albert Schweitzer.

There is a commonality.

When We See, We Truly See.

As we go along the path, we realize there is no one or only path.

If we are on a journey without beginning or end, where is there a need for a path?

Truth is a pathless land.

The greatest journeys are inward.

PRAYER

Pray well.

Always be in prayer.

It is a state of being.

It keeps you centered, calm and connected.

Pray for yourself.

Pray to yourself.

Pray for Others.

Pray to God.

You getting the idea, babe.

You are God.

Pray while breathing.

Pray while walking.

Pray while doing boom boom.

Pray while eenie meenie minie mo.

Pray while doing caca boom.

Pray while sitting.

Pray while standing.

Pray while walking.

Pray while working.

Pray while exercising.

Pray while relaxing.

Meditate on the Self, that be Yoreself, Pardner of Mine.

God lives in every part of Us.

Develop compassion for all animate and inanimate beings.

Be compassionate.

Pray well and prosper.

LOVE

- Friends
- Family
- Pets
- Charitable Activities
- Social Activities
- Work
- Religious Activities
- Spiritual Activities
- Sex
- Love
- Miscellaneous

HAPPINESS

- Sex
- Love
- Friends
- Family
- Pets
- Charitable Activities
- Social Activities
- Work
- Religious Activities
- Spiritual Activities
- Miscellaneous

RELIGIONS

- Hinduism
- Islam
- Christianity
- Buddhism
- Zoroastrianism
- Jainism
- Sikhism
- Jewism
- Animism
- Scientology
- Mormonism
- Bahai
- Folk Religions
- Miscellaneous

SPIRITUALITY

- Zen
- Taoism
- Confucianism
- Kabbala
- Vedanta
- Sufi Movement
- Bhakti Movement
- Yoga
- Animism
- Voodoo
- Miscellaneous

RELATIONSHIPS

- Relationship with self
- Relationship with family
- Relationship with friends
- Relationship with neighbors
- Relationship with neighborhoods
- Relationship with society
- Relationship with nation
- Relationship with world
- Relationship with universe
- Relationship with animate beings
- Relationship with inanimate beings
- Relationship with extraterrestrials
- Miscellaneous

COMPASSION

- Compassion
- Love
- Relatedness
- Empathy
- Forgiveness
- Miscellaneous

PRAYER

- Individual
- Group
- Connected
- Religious

- Spiritual
- Miscellaneous

Eat Well
Drink Well
Love Well & Be Happy
Sleep Well
Breathe Well & Be Mindful
Exercise Well
Work Well & Age Well
Do Sex Well
Sing, Do Music & Dance Well
Love Well & Be Well

ANATOMY AND PHYSIOLOGY

SKULL

This is a bony cage that protects the brain. It shapes the face. This is covered by skin, muscle and connective tissue. It spaces the eyes so we have stereoscopic vision. It spaces the ears so we can localize sounds in our environment. It has the maxilla and mandible that hold the teeth and are essential in eating and drinking.

It has a hole through which the spinal cord exits posteriorly, called the foramen magnum. It has areas where the eyes are lodged and can then connect to the brain at the back. It has openings for the nose and ears. It has openings for blood vessels and nerves which enter and exit this space.

When someone tries to conk us, thank god we have our skull to protect our most precious organ, the brain.

It contains the forebrain, midbrain and brainstem.

It contains vascular and neural structures running on the inside and outside of the skull.

The spinal cord exits through the foramen magnum along with its neurovascular components.

Trauma to these regions can cause pain and/or dysfunction.

Pressure on nerves and vessels supplying this region can cause pain and/or dysfunction.

Any process affecting the bone and/or internal contents can cause pain and/or dysfunction.

Inflammation, Infections, Ischemia, Trauma, Infiltrative processes, Cancer can cause pain and/or dysfunction.

BRAIN

It's good to have a brain. It is a huge supercomputer that directs our thoughts and lives. It is a beautifully designed organ. The brain and spinal cord form the central nervous system.

It consists of the forebrain, midbrain and hindbrain. There is grey matter and white matter in the brain. There are sulci and gyri on the surface of the brain. They have neurons and glial cells. We have motor, sensory and association areas.

Neurotransmitters include Glutamate, Gamma Aminobutyric Acid (GABA), Dopamine, Acetylcholine, Epinephrine, Norepinephrine, etc.

 The brain is enclosed by three membranes, Dura mater, Arachnoid mater and Pia mater. In between the Arachnoid mater and the Pia mater is the Cerebrospinal Fluid (CSF). The CSF circulating inside and outside the brain along with the spinal cord is all connected and maintained at a constant pressure. It is produced in the choroid plexuses and absorbed by the arachnoid granulations in the brain. It has nutritive, protective and waste removal functions.

The main areas of the brain are:

Cerebral hemispheres-right and left are connected by commissures including the corpus callosum. The cerebrum has the motor and sensory cortices in addition to association areas. The cortical areas are frontal, temporal, parietal and occipital ones. These have functional areas called Brodmann's areas. They control thought, sensation, etc.

Motor Cortex: Relays to brainstem and spinal regions.

- Frontal cortex
- Premotor cortex
- Supplementary motor cortex
- Primary somatosensory cortex
- Temporal cortex
- Parietal cortex
- Occipital cortex

Sensory Cortex: Peripheral relays to the brain.

- Visual cortex
- Auditory cortex
- Temporal cortex
- Insular cortex
- Somatosensory cortex

The frontal lobe subserves attention, abstract thinking, personality, behavior, etc.

The temporal lobe subserves speech, hearing, language, etc.

The parietal lobe subserves association, memory, etc.

The occipital lobe subserves vision, visual-spatial processing, etc.

The basal ganglia are nuclei which control behavior, movement control, etc.

The thalamus subserves relay functions, sensory processing, cognition, etc.

The hypothalamus subserves neuroendocrine regulation, autonomic nervous system regulation, circadian rhythms regulation, etc.

The cerebellum controls balance, coordination, motor control, etc.

The brainstem consists of the midbrain, pons and medulla which control various processes such as heart rate, respiration, sensory and motor control, etc.

Direct injury causes traumatic injury to multiple structures.

There is fluid in the enclosed ventricles of the brain and also surrounding the brain. The fluid outside is connected to the fluid inside. Fluid is always secreted and always absorbed. If there is a problem with these processes, we have volume, flow and/or pressure problems with attendant pathology.

It is intimately connected to multiple vascular structures.

It originates neural output to the special senses such as vision, smell and hearing.

It is affected by pressure and pain stimuli.

Aneurysms or Trauma can cause severe headaches.

Membranes in addition to fluid spaces can be involved in pathologic processes and cause pain and/or dysfunction.

Discrete neural, vascular and bony structures when involved can cause pain and/or dysfunction.

It is affected in central pain syndromes.

Inflammation, Infections, Ischemia, Trauma, Infiltrative processes, Cancer can cause pain and/or dysfunction.

Bacterial and/or Parasitic infections and/or related processes of the brain can cause pain and/or dysfunction.

Meningiomas, Glioblastoma Multiforme (GBM), etc are cancers that can cause pain and/or dysfunction.

Metastases from Breast, Lung, Skin Cancers, etc can cause pain and/or dysfunction.

SPINE

The spine consists of the spinal canal that transmits the spinal cord. The spinal cord has cervical, thoracic and lumbosacral areas which give out nerves innervating the extremities, viscera, etc. It is supplied by one anterior and two posterior spinal arteries.

The spinal areas have vertebrae, discs, facet joints, spinal nerves and multiple soft tissues acting in concert. Dysfunction of these structures, either individually or in concert, may cause structural, physiological and/or functional deficits. The ventral horns subserve mainly motor function while the posterior horns subserve sensory functions.

Ischemia or Infarction can cause severe functional deficits, usually due to cell injury or death.

Blockages in the pipes supplying blood to the spinal cord can cause ischemia and/or infarction.

Inflammation, Infiltration, Infection, Trauma, Cancer, etc can cause severe deficits in addition to pain and/or dysfunction.

HEART

The heart is a contractile muscular bag that pumps blood all over the body. It is organized into four chambers. It has its own blood supply subserved by the coronary arteries. It has multiple tubes that get blood in and out of the heart. It has its own paced electrical system.

The cells forming this structure are pacing cells, conductive cells and myocardial cells. The heart has an inner endocardium, middle myocardium and outer epicardium. The pericardium lines it on the outside.

The myocardium is very well supplied with blood, both from the lumina and the coronary arteries.

A pump that distributes oxygen and nutrients around the body using sets of pipes.

 Ischemia or Infarction can cause severe pain and/or dysfunction, usually due to cell injury or death.

Blockages in the pipes supplying blood to the heart can cause pain and/or dysfunction.

Heart valve pathologies can cause pain and/or dysfunction.

Inflammation, Infiltrative and Infective processes of the heart linings can cause pain and/or dysfunction.

Pericardial disease processes can cause pain and/or dysfunction.

Obstructions to the flow of blood to or from the heart can cause pain and/or dysfunction.

Decreased blood flow and resultant decreased oxygenation can cause tissue injury in the heart and/or associated structures that can cause pain and/or dysfunction.

LUNGS

The lungs are expansile structures, like bellows at an ironsmith, to help oxygenate blood and tissues. They have air sacs composed of cells that oxygenate our blood and remove carbon dioxide from our body. The air flows in through the trachea, bronchi and then progressively through smaller tubes till it gets to the alveoli that are like small balloons where air exchange takes place. Here, the oxygen is absorbed and carbon dioxide is expelled. The lungs are covered in pleural coverings.

The lining cells inside and outside the lung are sensitive structures and are painful to nociceptive and toxic inputs.

Ischemia can cause pain and/or dysfunction.

Hyperventilation and Hypoventilation, Hypoxic Injury, etc can affect the lungs and their sheaths, which can cause pain and/or dysfunction.

Trauma, Deposition Diseases, etc can cause pain and/or dysfunction with damage to multiple surfaces and/or structures.

Distension or Constriction of vascular structures can cause pain and/or dysfunction.

Inflammation, Injury or Infiltration of the pleural surfaces can cause pain and/or dysfunction.

Infective causes such as bacteria, fungi, mycobacteria, etc can cause pain and/or dysfunction.

Pulmonary Emboli, Granulomatosis, etc can cause pain and/or dysfunction.

Obstructive, Restrictive, Fibrotic processes can cause pain and/or dysfunction.

Cancers can cause pain and/or dysfunction, either primary or meta-static. Primary cancers are Small Cell Lung Carcinoma (SCLC) and Non Small Cell Lung Carcinomas (NSCLC).

Hypoxia from decreased oxygenation can cause tissue injury in the lung and/or surrounding structures that can cause pain and/or dysfunction.

LIVER

The liver is a metabolic factory that takes up and cleans toxins out of the blood. These can either be substances entering the bloodstream from the digestive tract or other organs-systems. It synthesizes proteins and also helps in digestion along with metabolism.

It secretes substances into the bile that help in digestion.

It synthesizes clotting factors that help in coagulation of the blood.

It helps in formation of hormones and in immunity.

It helps in inactivating and excreting drugs along with toxins.

Problems with the liver result in ineffective cleansing and increased nociception from these substances.

Internal and external coverings of the liver are nociceptive and their involvement can cause pain and/or dysfunction.

Inflammation, Infection, Ischemia, Trauma, Infiltrative processes, Cancer can cause pain and/or dysfunction.

Primary cancers of the liver are mainly HepatoCellular Carcinomas (HCC).

Dilatation or Constriction of their tubules can cause pain and/or dysfunction.

Budd-Chiari syndrome with blockage of the hepatic veins causes abdominal pain, ascites and liver enlargement.

Hepatitis and associated inflammation with organomegaly can cause pain and/or dysfunction.

PANCREAS

The pancreas is important in digestion, blood glucose control, endocrine functions, etc.

Ischemia, Infarcts, Infiltration, Cancer, Infection and Injury to tissue can cause pain and/or dysfunction.

Acute and chronic pancreatitis may cause pain and/or dysfunction.

Primary cancers of the pancreas are pancreatic adenocarcinomas, insulinomas, gastrinomas, etc.

Inflammation of the organ coverings can cause pain and/or dysfunction.

SPLEEN

This helps in blood cell production and filtering of the blood. It also functions as a cell reservoir. It has a significant role in the mononuclear phagocytic system.

It has an important function in immune modulation.

Ischemia, Infarcts, Infiltration, Infection, Cancer or Injury can cause pain and/or dysfunction.

Primary cancers of the spleen are hemangiomas and hemangiosarcomas.

Inflammation of the coverings can cause pain and/or dysfunction.

KIDNEYS

The kidneys are bags of cells that filter the blood and create urine. They also help in inactivating and excreting drugs and/or toxins.

They produce substances helpful in blood pressure control. They help maintain and regulate blood pressure, electrolyte balance, etc.

They are important for acid-base and osmolality control.

The kidneys are connected to the bladder through the ureters. The bladder drains to the outside through the urethra.

Renal tubules and the kidneys are susceptible to pain and/or dysfunction from distension.

Inflammation, Infection, Infiltration, Trauma and Cancer can cause pain and/or dysfunction.

Primary cancers of the kidneys are Wilms Tumor and Renal Cell Carcinoma (RCC).

Renal stones anywhere in the course of the genitourinary tract can cause pain and/or dysfunction.

Conditions affecting the coverings of the kidney can cause pain and/or dysfunction.

Dilatation, Obstruction and/or Constriction of the tubules and/or collecting regions can cause pain and/or dysfunction.

BLADDER

This is a collection device for urine before it is excreted. The bladder receives urine from the kidneys via the ureters and conveys it to the exterior via the urethra.

Distension can cause pain and/or dysfunction.

Inflammation or Infection of the bladder wall causes cystitis that can cause pain and/or dysfunction.

Infection, Infiltration, Trauma, Cancer of the bladder can cause pain and/or dysfunction.

Primary cancers of the bladder are mainly Transitional Cell Carcinomas (TCC).

Dyssynergia, Extrophy, Retention, etc can cause pain and/or dysfunction.

Increased intraluminal pressure can cause pain and/or dysfunction.

Conditions affecting the wall and/or linings of the bladder can cause pain and/or dysfunction.

PHARYNX, ESOPHAGUS, STOMACH, DUODENUM, SMALL & LARGE INTESTINES, SIGMOID COLON AND ANUS

The Gastrointestinal System (GI) is a tubular system for digesting and transporting food so we can get the energy we need to function. It has a significant role in Nutrition, Metabolism, Immunomodulation, etc.

UPPER GI TRACT

- Mouth
- Pharynx
- Esophagus
- Stomach
- Duodenum

SMALL INTESTINES

- Duodenum
- Jejunum
- Ileum

LARGE INTESTINES

- Cecum
- Appendix
- Ascending colon
- Transverse colon
- Descending colon
- Sigmoid colon
- Rectum
- Anus

Food is broken down into its constituents- simple sugars, amino acids and fatty acids.

The sugars are used in metabolism.

The amino acids are useful in body building.

The fatty acids are used for energy and/or stored and/or used in metabolic functions.

Distension or Constriction of the lumina can cause pain and/or structural and/or functional dysfunction.

Ulcers can cause pain and/or dysfunction.

Infections, Infiltration, Cancer can cause pain and/or dysfunction.

Cancers including Oropharyngeal cancer, Stomach cancer, Colorectal cancer, etc can cause pain and/or dysfunction.

Endometriosis, Gynecological problems, Post Surgical Scarring may affect the GI system and cause pain and/or dysfunction.

Noxious Stimuli, Ischemia, Trauma can cause pain and/or dysfunction.

Diverticulosis, Diverticulitis, Appendicitis, Inflammatory and/or Ulcerative Conditions can cause pain and/or dysfunction.

Infectious Conditions including amoebic, bacterial, viral, protozoal infections, etc can cause pain and/or dysfunction.

Conditions affecting the inner and outer linings or the walls of the intestines can cause pain and/or dysfunction.

UTERUS

It is a reproductive organ that helps in growing a baby. It has the capacity to supply blood and nutrients to the growing baby.

It is connected to the vagina through the cervix. The fundus is connected to the fallopian tubes. It has an inner endometrium, the middle myometrium and the outer perimetrium.

Inflammation, Trauma, Infiltration, Ischemia, Infection, etc can cause pain and/or dysfunction.

Fibroids, Adhesions, Cancer, etc can cause pain and/or dysfunction.

Conditions affecting the endometrial linings including bacterial and/or mycobacterial infections can cause pain and/or dysfunction.

ENDOMETRIUM

This lines the female reproductive tract, especially the uterus. It has a functional and a basal layer.

The vagina leads into the uterus. The uterus at its superolateral aspect has a fallopian tube on each side. The ovaries are on either side of the ends of the fallopian tubes. This literally opens up the abdominal cavity to the environment.

The endometrium can seed the peritoneum, and if and when these grow, they can cause severe pain and/or dysfunction from endometriosis.

Endometriosis can cause generalized and/or multiorgan involvement.

Endometritis, Endometriosis, Adenomyosis, Endometrial Hyperplasia, etc can cause pain and/or dysfunction.

This condition may need multiple surgeries to correct it, with varying levels of success. The surgeries and their postoperative sequelae in addition to the underlying conditions can cause pain and/or dysfunction.

Conditions affecting the linings of the genitourinary system can cause pain and/or dysfunction.

Distension, Infiltration, Ischemia, Infiltration, Infection, Trauma, Cancer, etc can cause pain and/or dysfunction.

Endometrial Cancer is the primary cancer and can cause pain and/or dysfunction.

OVARIES

The ovaries are the female equivalent of the testes. They create the ovum. It also has critical endocrine functions.

Ovarian cysts can cause pain and/or dysfunction.

Ovarian torsion with ischemia can cause severe pain and/or dysfunction.

Distension or Constriction can cause pain and/or dysfunction.

Infections, Infiltration, Trauma, Cancer or Inflammation can cause pain and/or dysfunction.

Primary cancers including ovarian cancer (OC), choriocarcinoma (CC), germ cell tumors (GCT), etc can cause pain and/or dysfunction.

Conditions affecting the linings can cause pain and/or dysfunction.

TESTES

The testicles are the male equivalent of the ovaries. They have reproductive and endocrine functions.

Torsion, Inflammation, Infiltration, Infection or Ischemia can cause pain and/or dysfunction.

Testicular Torsion, Testicular Rupture, Castration, etc are surgical emergencies.

Orchitis, Epididymitis, Varicocele, etc can cause pain and/or dysfunction.

Distention or Constriction of the tubular systems of the testes can cause pain and/or dysfunction.

Testicular Cancer (TC) can cause pain and/or dysfunction.

Conditions affecting the linings of the testes can cause pain and/or dysfunction.

EPIDIDYMIS

This is a structure on top of the testicle that connects it to the vas deferens. It has a head, body and tail.

Inflammation, Infection, Trauma, Infiltration or Ischemia can cause pain and/or dysfunction.

Epididymitis can be a very painful condition. It can cause additional structural and/or functional dysfunction.

This structure is present only in males.

PROSTATE

This is a gland around the urethra, which makes prostatic fluid in the ejaculate.

This structure is present only in males. The closest equivalent in women is the Skene's gland.

Infection, Infiltration, Cancer, Trauma or Inflammation can cause pain and/or dysfunction.

Benign Prostatic Hypertrophy (BPH) is a common condition affecting the prostate.

Prostatic Carcinoma (PC) is a common primary cancer which can cause pain, morbidity and/or mortality.

Prostatic Hypertrophy causes urinary flow and/or pressure problems along with superimposed conditions and/or affective states.

SPECIAL SENSES

The eyes are cameras that get us information of the world around us for seeing.

The ears are microphones that obtain auditory information around us for hearing.

The nostrils are sniffers that get us information on olfactory status or smell.

The tongue and oropharyngeal mucosa are tasters that subserve taste perception.

The auditory and vestibular systems of the ear subserve our balance functions.

Touch is usually subserved by pressure, vibration and joint sense.

Pain, heat and noxious stimuli are sensed by the cutaneous and mucosal systems.

Cancer can cause pain and/or dysfunction, either by primary or metastatic processes.

Inflammation, Ischemia, Infiltration, Infection, Trauma, etc can cause pain and/or dysfunction in the above mentioned systems, linings and spaces.

SPECIAL AREAS

Organs, Structures or Moieties not fitting into the classifications noted can cause pain and/or dysfunction based on altered states and/or physiologic alterations and/or pathologic processes either happening in them and/or their surroundings.

We can diagnose, problem solve and fix them.

The same thinking patterns, analysis and action pathways are utilized as delineated above.

BONES

Bones are structures that hold us up, protect organs and structures, are mineral repositories, enable motion etc.

Bones are covered on the outer surface by the periosteum and on the inner surface by the endosteum.

Bones have a cavity inside called the marrow. The main types of mineralized tissue are cortical and cancellous bone. Bones contain osteoblasts and osteoclasts.

Bones are very important in protective, structural, mineral homeostasis, acid-base balance functions, sequestration of toxic substances, endocrine functions, etc.

Bone per se has no pain receptors and is thought to be insensitive to pain.

Periosteum and endosteum are sensitive to pain.

Bone marrow is important in formation of cellular elements of the blood.

Conditions affecting the periosteum or endosteum can cause pain and/or dysfunction.

Conditions affecting the cortical structures or marrow can cause pain and/or dysfunction.

Integrity disruptions or fractures can cause pain and/or dysfunction.

Osteoarthritis, Osteoporosis, Joint disorders, etc can cause pain and/or dysfunction.

Ankylosing Spondylitis (AS) and other similar restrictive conditions can cause pain and/or dysfunction.

Resorptive conditions can cause pain and/or dysfunction.

Infection, Inflammation, Infiltration, Infection, Trauma, Cancer, etc can cause pain and/or dysfunction.

Primary bone cancers like Osteosarcoma, Osteoblastoma etc can cause pain and/or dysfunction.

Primary cancers elsewhere with metastases to bone such as Breast, Prostate, Lung, Kidney, etc can cause pain and/or dysfunction.

Leukemia, Multiple Myeloma (MM), Hodgkin's disease, Paget's disease, etc can cause pain and/or dysfunction.

Deposition Diseases including Calcium Pyrophosphate Deposition Disease (CPPD) and/or similar conditions can cause pain and/or dysfunction.

Osteomalacia can cause pain and/or dysfunction.

Fluorosis and/or congenital bone disorders and/or syndromes can cause pain and/or dysfunction.

MUSCLES

Muscles are structures composed of contractile proteins, actin and myosin, that connect bones and tissues.

Muscles help us in moving around, maintain posture, perform actions, help power our heart, help power our intestines, visceral functions, etc. There are over 650 plus muscle sets.

We have skeletal, cardiac and smooth muscles. We have voluntary and involuntary muscles. We have Type I and Type II fibers.

We use aerobic and anaerobic metabolism in the functioning of this system.

They allow movement and function throughout the body.

Trauma, Inflammation, Infection, Infiltration and Ischemia can cause pain and/or dysfunction.

Neuromuscular Disorders (NMD) can cause spasticity, contractures, disordered function, etc including immobility and/or paralysis.

Primary Muscle Disorders can cause spasticity, contractures, disordered function including dystonias and/or paralysis.

Distension and Contractures can cause pain and/or dysfunction.

Cancer can cause pain and/or dysfunction, either through primary or metastatic processes.

SKIN

The skin is a sheet covering the whole body. This is a barrier that protects us and gives us temperature regulation, protection from the environment, homeostasis, temperature regulation, sensation, synthesis of vitamin D, absorption, etc.

It has sweat glands which help us in temperature regulation. We have hair that helps both in temperature regulation and has immense cosmetic benefits.

It consists of the epidermis, dermis and subcutaneous fat, all with their unique structures and functions.

It allows us to interact with our environments.

It can be painful from Traumatic, Ischemic, Infective, Infiltrative or Inflammatory processes.

Cancer, either primary or metastatic, can cause pain and/or dysfunction.

Melanoma, Basal Cell Carcinoma (BCC), Squamous Cell Carcinoma (SCC), Merkel Cell Carcinoma (MCC), etc need to be closely monitored and managed with an emphasis on recognizing, evaluating and treating them early.

Contractures can cause pain and/or dysfunction.

Pigmented skin is more resistant to skin damage but care should be taken as with fair skinned individuals to regulate the amount of skin exposure to either the sun and/or light stress.

Pigmented skin is more prone to Keloids after surgery and/or trauma, stretch marks from pregnancy, etc.

Pigmented skin can still get cancer easily from sun and/or light exposure which needs to be kept in mind when evaluating for carcinomatous processes affecting the skin.

FASCIAE

These are like plastic sheets that encapsulate muscles and organs. They are connective tissue sheaths.

They separate muscles, organs, structures, etc in our bodies.

They are classified as superficial, deep, parietal and visceral depending on location and function.

Fascial compartments are well delineated and seen in both the upper and lower limbs.

Fascial sheets can become painful from Inflammatory, Ischemic, Infiltrative and/or Traumatic processes.

Post Trauma, fascial compartments may become massively pressurized and this may be a surgical emergency. The pressure needs to be relieved with decompression to help prevent tissue necrosis and/or death.

Cancer-primary and/or metastatic processes can cause pain and/or dysfunction.

VISCERA

Visceral structures, whether in the thorax or abdomen, have distinctive structures, coverings, nerves and vascular supply. These are in turn covered by bony, muscular, fascial and skin structures.

All these structures when affected can cause pain and/or dysfunction.

We need to correctly delineate what is aberrant or abnormal, problem solve and then work on fixing it.

Problem solving skills that we have developed as noted above would help in diagnosing, decision making and management or rectification of solitary and/or multiple and/or any problems. Unique features and physiologies of each particular area and/or system need to be kept in mind and considered when looking at discrete systems and subsystems in our bodies.

MICROBIOME

All the bacteria, viruses, fungi, bacteriophages, protozoa, archaea, etc that colonize, seed and live on our skin, in the intestines, on the mucosal surfaces of reproductive organs, etc constitute our microbiome. This important "Organ", about 200 trillion organisms worth, helps in regulation of immunity, helps nourish cells, helps digestion in addition to innumerable other functions that are constantly being elucidated.

They live consensually with us and modulate our immunity and our wellbeing. We are still in the learning process of how exactly this whole new system or organ influences us and our health. This vast system is very important for our health and wellbeing. Our genes, immune system and body may be self modulating and working intimately together with this immense living shield. It is a mutually beneficial symbiotic relationship.

It has about 200 times the genetic material we all have in our bodies. We may have been swapping gene and nucleotide segments with our microbiome which in fact enriches us. Guess how much our microbiome weighs? About five pounds per person! Wow!

It is a great idea to eat prebiotics and prebiotics to help our lil friends flourish. They flourish, we flourish and we are healthy.

ENERGY

We are all made of electric and magnetic force fields. Cell metabolism is intrinsically electromagnetic in nature. If we use special cameras, we can image these force fields. Electricity flows through us and each electric field has its own heat and electromagnetic signatures. Once we can sense, we can also map energy. Once we map energy, we can look to add and/or take away and/or modulate it. This may have wide applications for diagnosing and/or rectifying physiologic and/or pathologic conditions affecting living systems now and in the near future.

***

We are Energy.

Universe is Energy.

God is Energy.

***

What Is The Prime Directive?

Know the Problem?

Know the Problem?

Know the Problem?

***

What is the problem?

Where is the problem?

What is the extent of the problem?

What do we know?

What do we not know?

What do we need to know?

How shall we get what we need to know?

What shall we do?

What are our options?

What options do we like?

What options don't we like?

How shall we do what we want to do?

***

Think!!!

Analyze!!!

Act!!!

DIAGNOSTIC TESTING

IMAGING

- X-RAY
- COMPUTED TOMOGRAPHY (CT)
- MAMMOGRAPHY
- ULTRASOUND (US)
- ELASTOGRAPHY
- DUPLEX VENOUS SCANNING
- DIGITAL SUBTRACTION ANGIOGRAPHY (DSA)
- MAGNETIC RESONANCE ANGIOGRAPHY (MRA)
- FUNCTIONAL MAGNETIC RESONANCE IMAGING (fMRI)
- MAGNETIC RESONANCE IMAGING (MRI)
- SCINTIGRAPHY
- SINGLE PHOTON EMISSION COMPUTED TOMOGRAPHY (SPECT)
- POSITRON EMISSION TOMOGRAPHY (PET)
- PHOTOACOUSTIC IMAGING
- OPTOACOUSTIC IMAGING
- FUNCTIONAL NEAR INFRARED SPECTROSCOPY
- MAGNETIC PARTICLE IMAGING
- ELECTRICAL IMPULSE TOMOGRAPHY

- DIFFUSE OPTICAL TOMOGRAPHY
- RETINAL SCANNING
- NUCLEAR MEDICINE TESTING
- OPHTHALMOLOGICAL TESTING
- SPECIALISED TESTING
- MISCELLANEOUS

METABOLIC TESTING

- SMA-7
- SMA-18
- LIVER FUNCTION TESTS (LFT)
- KIDNEY OR RENAL FUNCTION TESTS (RFT)
- SPECIALIZED METABOLIC TESTING
- CARDIAC METABOLITES TESTING
- PROSTATE TESTING
- THYROID FUNCTIONAL TESTING (TFT)
- RHEUMATOLOGIC TESTING
- AUTO IMMUNE DISEASE TESTING
- HEMATOLOGIC TESTING
- PROTEIN ELECTROPHORESIS
- HORMONAL TESTING
- TOXICOLOGY TESTING
- SPECIALISED TESTING
- MISCELLANEOUS

MICROBIOLOGY TESTING

- BLOOD CULTURES
- URINE CULTURES
- CEREBROSPINAL FLUID (CSF) TESTING

- CULTURE/SENSITIVITIES
- INFECTIVE AGENT TESTING
- SPECIALISED TESTING
- MISCELLANEOUS

PATHOLOGY TESTING

- MOLECULAR TESTING
- CANCER TESTING
- PAP SCREENING
- TISSUE BIOPSY TESTING
- IMMUNOLOGIC TESTING
- CELLULOMICS TESTING
- ANTIGENIC TESTING
- SPECIALISED TESTING
- MISCELLANEOUS

FUNCTIONAL TESTING

- ELECTROENCEPHALOGRAPHY
- ELECTROMYOGRAPHY
- EVOKED POTENTIALS
- NEUROGRAPHY
- CENTRAL NERVOUS SYSTEM TESTING
- PERIPHERAL NERVOUS SYSTEM TESTING
- SYMPATHETIC SYSTEM TESTING
- PARASYMPATHETIC SYSTEM TESTING
- PULMONARY FUNCTION TESTING
- CARDIAC FUNCTION TESTING
- VASCULAR SYSTEM TESTING
- GASTROINTESTINAL TESTING

- MODIFIED BARIUM SWALLOW
- UROLOGIC TESTING
- GENITAL SYSTEM TESTING
- RENAL TESTING
- ADRENAL TESTING
- LOCOMOTORY FUNCTION TESTING
- MISCELLANEOUS

NUCLEIC ACID AND PROTEIN TESTING

- POLYMERASE CHAIN REACTION TESTING
- REVERSE TRANSCRIPTION POLYMERASE CHAIN REACTION
- RNA SEQUENCING
- PROTEOME SEQUENCING
- METABOLOMICS
- CELLULOMICS
- EXOME SEQUENCING
- WHOLE GENOME SEQUENCING
- MISCELLANEOUS

WEIGHT MANAGEMENT STRATEGIES AND SURGICAL OPTIONS

What are the options for a person with weight or body asymmetry problems? Let's look at them in more detail. Once we know our options, it is much easier to decide which option is right for us. It sets us free. Always discuss all options with your doctor or healthcare professional.

WHAT IF WE DO NOTHING?

It is an option. Things can get better; Things can get worse. Watchful waiting may be a good option in some circumstances.

For acute issues, if you can wait for it to resolve, wait? Perform diagnostics as needed to get the most information about the condition.

For chronic issues, it might be good to check what is causing it and then look at all the options available and then choose the option that makes the most sense to you.

EATING BETTER

As we see ourselves eating better, we eat better.

Eat in small portions.

Eat mindfully.

Eat with gratitude.

We have multiple feedback loops between our bodies, our hormonal axes and our brain circuits that control our intake and output. Be in balance.

Have smart snacks and in moderation.

Drink abundant quantities of water.

Let fiber be your friend.

Eliminate toxins well.

Source and get the best help and advice as needed.

Love your life.

Enjoy!!!

EXERCISE & MANUAL THERAPIES

We can exercise on our own making sure we don't reinjure the affected region.

We can do physical therapy

We can train with an athletic trainer

We can work with a chiropractor.

We can do massage therapy

We can do Yoga

We can do Pilates.

We can Walk.

We can work out at a gym or health club.

We can use specialized equipment to exercise discrete areas.

We can use either wet or dry saunas. The heat helps with the pain. It raises our metabolic rate helping us feel better and burn more calories. It can be a social event too. Please do use Finnish, Turkish and Russian saunas if you have access.

If you have snow or live in hot deserts and you don't have access to safe, clean exercise spaces, head out to your nearest mall, department store or any big retailer or public space. The space is usually warm or cooled and clean. It's a beautiful place to shake your stuff, walk and exercise. If you buy something, it's great for the economy. If not, it's great to look and enjoy.

We can do aquatic therapy. Because we don't have that much weight in water and because it cushions us, we can exercise the spine or involved joints with decreased risk of injury. It helps us negate the effects of gravity and helps promote pain free movements.

Use a pool frequently, at least a few times a week. It's a great and relaxing exercise option. You can do it at your own pace. It gives you good cardiovascular conditioning. It's great for relaxation. The water helps support our weight and we can exercise better and longer reducing the effects of gravity on our joints and body. This helps prevent wear and tear on our joints-muscles, keeps them and us healthier and happier in the long run.

Walk in Water. Run in Water. Exercise in Water. Do Martial Arts in Water. Do Jazz Aerobics in Water. Dance in Water. Sing in Water. Do Cardio in Water. Do Weight Lifting in Water. Do Calisthenics. Do Gymnastics. Do Anything you like, Do Sex in Water. Enjoy!.

BEHAVIORAL, PSYCHOLOGICAL AND PSYCHIATRIC SERVICES

This is a very important component of a comprehensive Weight Management program. Sometimes, we are right on target and focused. Sometimes, we may need help to change our thinking, our projections, our mental constructs, our motivations and behaviors, our fears and phobias, our reward options, physical-mental-spiritual well being and homeostasis, etc. We need to access the best information. We need to access the best providers. We need to meld this into a program that works best for us. Please access behavioral therapists, dieticians, wellness coaches, life coaches, psychologists, psychotherapists, medical providers, psychiatrists, etc for obtaining the most helpful resources for YOU.

Lifestyle management, Lifestyle modification, Virtual gastric bands, Virtual weight modeling, Virtual volumetrics, Anxiety management, Insightful therapies, Meditation, Yoga, Cognitive Behavioral Therapy, Acceptance and Commitment Therapy, Hypnosis, etc may all play a critical role in Weight Management.

- Do a comprehensive analysis.
- Form a detailed mental image of where you are and where you want to be.
- Visualize the start and end points.
- Form a realistic strategy
- Write down a fully fleshed, well planned strategy.
- Put down smart, implementable goals.

- Target small steps on your journey.
- Accomplish each step.
- Reward yourself for each success.
- Celebrate each success.
- Small failures or setbacks are okay.
- Do not beat yourself up for failure.
- Chuck failures into a virtual dustbin.
- Maintain accurate logs.
- Winning and Losing are two sides of the same coin. They are both Illusions of the Mind. Transcend the opposites and WIN.
- Rigorous execution is key.
- Enlist support of friends and family.
- Go on your journey in Gratitude.
- Go on your journey in Peace.
- Follow The Living Sutras.
- Eat Smart and Be SuperSlim.
- Be Active and Be SuperSlim.
- Think Smart and Be SuperSlim.
- Do Smart and Be SuperSlim
- Be Happy and Be SuperSlim.
- Think Yourself SuperSlim.
- Become SuperSlim.
- Yay. You Win. We Win. We All Win. Enjoy!!!
- Access the best knowledge banks, resources, therapists as needed. What you need is what you need. Let go of the negatives. Focus on the positives. You and your healthcare team know what is best for YOU.
- LIVE WELL. LIVE SMART. LIVE HAPPY.

MEDICATIONS

Your doctors may consider using different kinds of medications to targeted different mechanisms of action or systems.

Food is a drug. Control your food intake smartly. Use timed protocols.

Your doctors may consider using appetite suppressants to help control appetite and reduce food intake.

Your doctors may consider using catecholamine releasing agents for their appetite suppressant actions.

Your doctors may consider using medications that reduce or prevent absorption of different food groups or nutrients such as Orlistat.

Your doctors may consider using hormonal enhancers or declinators.

Your doctors may consider using psychotropic medications as needed for these disorders

Your doctors may consider using Anorectics.

Your doctors may consider using fiber supplements to induce satiety, bulk up stools and lowering caloric absorption.

A wide range of other medications and molecules are currently being evaluated worldwide and may be used as per medical recommendations.

We can also use emerging technologies such as genomics, transcriptomics, proteomics, cellulomics or nanomedicine to devise path breaking biologics solutions.

COMPLEMENTARY AND ALTERNATIVE MEDICINE (CAM)

There is modern medicine. There is complementary medicine. There is alternative medicine. There is not only one stream or one branch of medicine. These are different parts of one whole system designed to ameliorate, help cure diseases and dysfunction of the human body.

Let us learn from anything and everything. What we know is a miniscule fraction of all the knowledge available in the universe. We have millions of plants, animals, species, etc waiting to be discovered, catalogued and studied. Let's not close ourselves to what we can learn now and in the future. The following few are representative but are not a full list of care options.

Consider Acupuncture: An ancient Chinese technique involving needles and/or knives to work on the energy channels of the body.

Consider Homeopathy: This initially originated in Germany and then spread worldwide. Minute amounts of a drug are given to cause opposite effects in the body.

Consider Ayurveda: It is an ancient healing art from India. It uses a lot of plants, inorganic products such as bhasmas, etc. It tries to balance the three main doshas or life forces in our bodies. It aims for balance. The practitioners mainly look to diagnose from pulse reading, oral examination, etc.

Look for excellent quality and well trained, authentic practitioners. Use products and services with world class standards.

Consider various other options based on common sense, need and implement smartly!!!

ANTIAGING MEDICINE (AAM)

With antiaging technologies, we can slow down or reverse multiple metabolic processes.

We can use smart exercise regimens to slow down these processes and their effects.

We can use nutritional supplementation in addition to food to help modulate body function..

We can use specialized pharmaceuticals and/or nutraceuticals and/or metabolic extracts like Metformin, Thymosin, etc for specific effects.

We can use disc decompression, manual therapies, manipulation under anesthesia, hyperbaric oxygen therapy, etc to help modify specific processes and/or reverse discrete pathology.

We can use emerging technologies such as genomics, transcriptomics, proteomics, cellulomics or nanomedicine.

IMPLANTABLE GASTRIC STIMULATION

Implantable gastric stimulation involves stimulation of the external surface of the stomach which is thought to stimulate the enteric circuits and induce a feeling of satiety. It is not as effective currently as other bariatric procedures but may show promise in the future with better implants, materials and techniques.

We can use newer technologies including Nanotechnology, Materials Science with new Smart Materials, Robotics, Artificial Intelligence, Internet of Things, etc to fashion newer arrays-instrumentation platforms for better functions and uses.

INTERVENTIONAL, MINIMALLY INVASIVE, ROBOTIC AND SURGICAL PROCEDURES

GASTROPLASTY

This can either be a vertical banded gastroplasty, gastric banding, sleeve gastrectomy, etc. This surgery involves reducing the volume of the stomach. Intragastric and/or Extragastric balloons, Gastric plication, etc are viable alternatives with similar mechanisms of action.

GASTRIC BYPASS

Roux-en-Y Gastric bypass, sleeve gastrectomy with duodenal switch, etc lead to restriction of absorption, malabsorption and alterations in gut hormones.

ADDITIONAL SURGERY AND SERVICES

Biliopancreatic diversion, Biliopancreatic diversion with duodenal switch, Jejunoileal bypass, Endoluminal sleeve, etc. help block absorption of food.

Additional plastic surgery and/or other medical-surgical specialty services can be provided for optimization of function and structure in these populations. Multidisciplinary teams are of great help in comprehensive provision of any and all needed services. Use wisely and as needed.

RISKS & BENEFITS OF INTERVENTIONAL AND/OR SURGICAL CARE

BENEFITS

- Weight Loss
- Amelioration of Disease Conditions
- Reversal of Disease Conditions
- Problem Relief
- Problem Cessation
- Functional Gains
- Decreased Medication Usage
- Return to Work & Leisure Activities
- Increased Longevity
- Miscellaneous

RISKS AND COMPLICATIONS

- Surgical risks
- Infection
- Anesthesia Complications
- Wound Care Issues
- Vascular Injury
- Lymphatic Injury
- Post Operative Adhesions
- Hyperparathroidism
- Hyperoxaluria
- Rhabdomyolosis
- Renal Disorders
- Gastrointestinal Disorders
- Adrenal Disorders

- Reproductive Issues
- Hormonal Issues
- Pyschiatric Issues
- Morbidity
- Mortality
- Death
- Miscellaneous

HEALTHCARE AND TECHNOLOGY

Health is a basic human need. It is something to be treasured. Sometimes, we don't juggle our priorities and wind up with an unsatisfactory system. Well, we can always work to get it back in top fettle. Our perspectives on this are that we can work to make anything better. There is only one way of doing it, and that's the right way. Let us embark on this journey together.

We all love to sing the praises of modern medicine in prolonging longevity. However, the main things that have contributed to this are the implementation and provision of hygiene, clean water-air-food, indexed with public health measures such as sewerage, environmental engineering, social engineering, vaccinations and widespread health coverage. If we couple these with well-trained providers, good facilities and cutting edge technologies, we have the best chance of making it work. We believe a lot of countries in our era have some of the best knowledge banks and care technologies in the world. These are being aggressively rolled out across to prevent disease and promote health. Every nation needs to join in and lead. As this is an interconnected world, diseases or conditions affecting one part of the world soon affect everyone, everywhere as we are seeing in the 2019-20 coronavirus pandemic. We need to collaborate, share knowledge and best technologies-practices so we keep learning in real time.

We think it is great to have well trained doctors. When they see a patient, they look for patterns. They like to see what is known. They like to see what is unknown. If they have an idea, that's great. If they don't, that's great too. If they need other doctors to help, they get that done as soon as possible. Then they look to see if they can help effectively. It is good to make sure there is a point person-provider-institution to control and manage this process. A good primary care physician and proper specialists are all necessary in a balanced health team. Any known diagnostics that are needed to get to know fully and precisely, they need to get done. Once they have a good idea about the process, they go over the available options. Whatever the patient and their provider agree on is always the best option and they can then proceed smartly. It is better not to do things that the patient doesn't want. It is better not to do something the patient wants but that they don't agree with medically or in keeping with best practices. Being smart and reasonable is a key requirement all around.

Artificial Intelligence is going to radically reshape life and healthcare both in our lifetimes and in the future. We can also use information technology (IT), Machine Learning (ML), Machine Vision (MV), Internet of Things (IOT), Data Mining (DM), Cloud Computing (CC) and other emerging technologies to refashion healthcare, delivery, monitoring, diagnostics and precision therapeutics. This will allow us to fundamentally change our understanding and provision of smart care.

People are responsible for their choices. We eat sensibly. We exercise. We do preventive care. We play sports. We get involved in community. We smile. We work. We play. We pay for our care and our health before paying for newer wheels for the car or a nice vacation. We are responsible. Period. We pay for care, whether it is us or us making sure our insurance or care provider does. If we don't, such is life. You get what you pay for. The buck really stops with you. Responsibility is empowering.

We need to invest more in preventive medicine now. We need to make people and providers responsible and responsive in their care. Doctors and hospitals need to reasonably price care. Governments or insurance companies should be made to pay for needed care. Everyone needs to be made responsible for their course and decisions. Healthier Systems, Healthier People, Healthier World.

A clinical consultation costs about 10 dollars in India or Asia versus 100-500 dollars in America or Europe.

Quality heart or spine surgery usually costs around 5,000-20,000 dollars in India versus 50,000-100,000 dollars in USA.

Knee or hip surgery costs 5,000-10,000 dollars in India versus 30,000-50,000 in America.

A hip, knee or spine implant-hardware may cost between 300-1,000 dollars in India versus 20,000-50,000 dollars in USA. The making costs are usually under 200 dollars in Asia.

A hospital bed per night for an admitted patient in India costs around 100 dollars versus easily over 1,000 dollars in USA or Europe. What a difference! What savings! What opportunities!

A caesarean section costs about 30,000-50,000 dollars at a top hospital in America and about 3,000-7,000 dollars at a top hospital in India. The care is similar or better in India. Look at the difference. We need to start marketing care in India all over the world so we can be a resource for everyone and attract tens of millions of patients. It's time to market fully worldwide and dominate entire sectors and industries. Employment opportunities in the Millions!!!

A state of the art ventilator, 1,000-7,000 dollars in India versus 25,000-50,000 dollars in America or Europe. Similar cost savings are seen in monitors, hospital beds, ultrasound machines, personal protective equipment, diagnostics, vaccines, medications, services, etc.

It's very similar for most other procedures, interventions, surgery, laboratory and medical care. We need to unleash rapid innovation worldwide and use the best products-services at reasonable prices. It's time to open up healthcare at the best prices and quality all over the world and/or open up access worldwide to areas doing the best job at the best price like India, Thailand, Korea, etc.

With the current pandemic, we hear of companies rapidly innovating, solving problems and coming up with new devices, products and services. We think it is great to involve smart, engaged people everywhere, let them innovate-collaborate-problem solve and prototype path breaking products-solutions-services. Use disruption as a positive force. Embrace the new. Think!!!

- Dyson, the vacuum company, makes a new smart ventilator in about a week.
- DRDO in India in conjunction with public and private companies makes a smart ventilator in about three weeks that can ventilate 4-8 patients at a time. This costs around 6,000-8,000 dollars.
- AgVa Healthcare in India makes artificial intelligence enabled ventilators costing about 1,000-4,000 dollars.
- Multiple Indian public and private entities, defence labs, universities make ventilators, oxygen concentrators, sanitizing units, sanitizers, bio isolation gear, etc.
- Companies in different countries retool to make personal protective equipment including masks, face shields, etc. It increases self reliance and preparedness.
- Multiple start ups, Non profits, NGO's, Empowered Groups, etc. make simple ventilators that they open source and share worldwide.
- Different vaccine groups worldwide are collaborating and sharing information in real time while coming up with vaccine candidates.

- Convention centers, community spaces, repurposed buildings, etc. are converted into field hospitals with hospital like facilities, quarantine units, etc. This massively expands healthcare capacity and outreach to people in various countries.
- People using technology like Arogya Setu in India to get real time information on risk factors, health status, exposure, etc.
- Multiple countries working together and with the World Health Organization are fighting jointly against this global pandemic.
- Millions of healthcare personnel volunteering all over to help their communities, countries and the world.
- Multiple nations donating and sharing ventilators, protective equipment, knowledge bases, supply chains, healthcare personnel, etc. to countries needing assistance.

With newer technologies including Telediagnostics, Telemonitoring, Telemedicine, Artificial Intelligence, Machine Learning, Robotic Surgery, etc; it is easier to access the best and most viable resources worldwide. These are great for consultations, procedures, surgery, medical and/or continuing care. Preventive Medicine, Proper Diagnostics, Fantastic Algorithms, Timely Interventions, Precision Medicine, Best Care; These all make for a Better World.

India has started a huge healthcare program called Ayushman Bharat for providing free access and comprehensive medical-surgical care to about 500 million people. This costs about 5 Lakhs or under $7000 per family per year. This covers people who are traditionally too poor or unable to access care. It covers all care, diagnostics, medical treatment and surgery at any hospital, government or private, for those enrolled in the system, anywhere over the entire country of India. Full portability of medical coverage and medical care is assured. Big data, data mining, digitized records and cutting edge information technology is used to run this program. It removes access to care and prevents serious illness from bankrupting entire families.

Let us give Ayushman Bharat (AB) or Universal Healthcare (UH) for Below Poverty Level (BPL) families in India, government employees, armed forces, central forces, state forces, etc. It's also time to offer it on a payment basis to any and all Indians who want to enroll so it really becomes Universal Healthcare (UH) for all Indians. Government is Payor. Private Sector is Provider. We can leverage people, tech and smarts for the best healthcare in India and World. Let's do millions of healthcare start ups in India. Let us start millions of healthcare manufacturing units in India. Let us start millions of healthcare service companies in India. It is now time to become numero uno in healthcare fields worldwide.

We can easily generate 10 to 20 million new Indian jobs in the Healthcare Sector by 2025. We use these trained personnel to provide world class care for our massive population of 1.3 billion people. Once we do in India, we can then roll out worldwide for countries that may benefit. There are massive opportunities for all of us with immense benefits. We get to improve our healthcare infrastructure, personnel availability and care provision. Let us get it on and start investing in and for ourselves today. Let us be a light unto the nations of the world. Let us disassociate healthcare access and outcomes from personal affluence and/or national wealth and/or resources.

We need to start taking care of our societies and our most vulnerable individuals. Let us get everyone fed, clothed, educated, empowered and healthy in India and Worldwide. It has certainly become much better but it is good to intervene locally-regionally-globally and fix all the problems we can.

Open systems are good. They are good in technology. They are good in medicine. They are good in society. As all good systems go, everything starts at home. We are open in our families, our interactions, our lives.

As we are open, we do not need to hide. Hiding creates stress. Some of the fruits of this will be sweet. Some of the fruits of this will be painful. Once we decide that either is good, we are already free. Once we are free, we are in truth. Once we are in truth, we are in god. Once we are in truth, what need do we have to be afraid?

Once we are free, we are free to ask. Ask things of ourselves and of others. Push the envelope. We are free in relationships. We are free in life. Freedom ennobles us.

Once we start in our personal sphere, we move on to our neighborhoods and society. We make them better. We expect great things of ourselves. We expect great things of others. Once we expect great things, great things happen. If they do, that's great. If they don't, well, let's make it happen.

We then go on to nations and the world. Open systems. Open from outside. Open from inside. Open everywhere. Open between people. Open between people and government. Open with consequences. This is disruptive. Disruption is inevitable. Disruption is good. Embrace disruption continually. Nothing is inherently good or bad. It depends on how we use the process to lead the search for truth.

Blockchain, Internet of Things, Machine Learning, Machine Vision, Artificial Intelligence, Deep Tech, Information Technology, Smart Analytics, Smart Surveillance, Cloud Computing, 5G Tech, etc will fundamentally rewire our lives and lead to astounding leaps in technology, safety and effectiveness, Yay. A much better life waits for us in the near future.

None of this is going to be easy. Easy is never good. If we get things too easy, we would never get to our full potential. Adversity challenges us. Adversity shapes us. We should always go look for adversity if it doesn't come seeking us. Once we start on the path, the path always leads onwards.

We can then reshape society in our image. It may go the way we want it to. It may not. As we have said before, both are good. Once we transcend the pairs of opposites, we are in truth. Truth Always Wins.

We have great people. We have great systems. We have great societies. We have great nations. We have a great world. We can always make or have a great world. We are truly great.

What problems can we delineate?

How can we quantify them?

What solutions can we come up with?

How can we implement these in a timely and sensible manner?

How can we track progress and tweak solutions in real time?

How can we all win?

RESOURCE GUIDE

Adult BMI Calculator

www.cdc.gov

Pediatric BMI Calculator

www.cdc.gov/healthyweight/bmi/calculator.html

Obesity Society

www.obesity.org

International Federation for the Surgery of Obesity and Metabolic Disorders

www.ifso.com

American Society for Metabolic and Bariatric Surgery

www.asmbs.org

International Society of Aesthetic Plastic Surgery

www.isaps.org

American Diabetes Association

www.diabetes.org

Calorie Restriction Society

www.calorierestriction.org

United States Department of Agriculture

www.usda.gov

American Heart Association

www.americanheart.org

American Cancer Society

www.cancer.org

Centers for Disease Control

www.cdc.gov

National Institutes of Health

www.nih.gov

Food and Drug Administration

www.fda.gov

National Sleep Foundation

www.sleepfoundation.org

Mayo Clinic

www.mayoclinic.com

Johns Hopkins

www.hopkinsmedicine.org

American College of Physicians

www.acponline.org

World Health Organization

www.who.int

Apollo Hospitals

www.apollohospitals.com

Bumrungrad International Hospital

www.bumrungrad.com/en

Massachusetts Institute of Technology

www.mit.edu

National University of Singapore

www.nus.edu

Peking University

www.english.pku.cn

Sorbonne Universite

www.sorbonne-universite.fr

Oxford University

www.ox.ac.uk

ABOUT THE AUTHOR

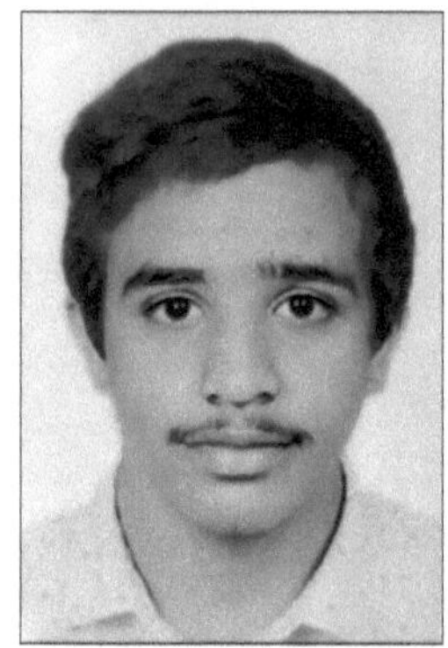

K Abhishek Reddy completed his Bachelors in Business Administration from Bharathiar University in Telangana, India. He has execu-
tive and leadership experience in the Food and Hospitality business.
In addition, he takes a keen interest in health, fitness and sports. He
is an avid public speaker and health advocate.

ABOUT THE AUTHOR

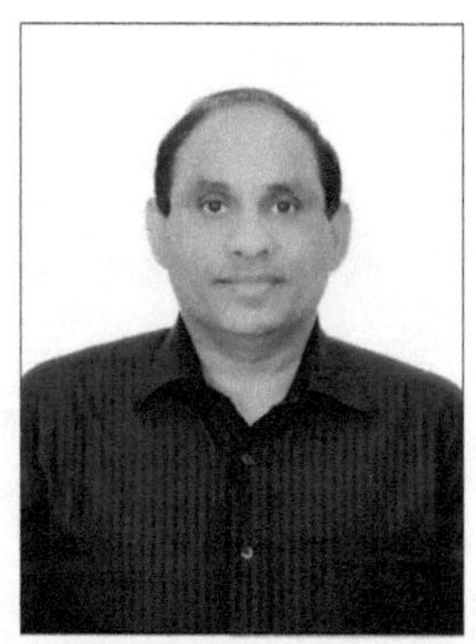

K. Mahesh Reddy, MD was accepted into the top medical schools in India at the relatively young age of 17. He has completed his medical training and graduated from Gandhi Medical College in Hyderabad, India. He went on to complete his Residency from Temple University Hospital, Temple University, Philadelphia, Pennsylvania in Physical Medicine and Rehabilitation. He completed a Fellowship in Pain Management from University Hospitals of Cleveland, Case Western Reserve University in Cleveland, Ohio. He has been accepted at the most prestigious institutions both in India and America. He has presented extensively in both the national and international arenas. His interests include Precision Medicine, Genomics and Deep Tech.